PICKLEBALL POWER:

A Comprehensive Guide to Staying Healthy and Fit for Peak Performance

By **Steve Jordan**, BS, CSCS, PES, CES, CPT, HLC

Peak Performance and Fitness Coach

<u>Disclaimer:</u>

The information provided in this book, "Pickleball Power," is for educational and informational purposes only. The author is not liable for any injury, loss, or damage incurred as a result of following the techniques, exercises, or advice presented herein. Readers are advised to consult with a qualified instructor or medical professional before attempting any physical activity or implementing any strategies discussed in this book.

<u>Liability Clause:</u>

By engaging in any activities, exercises, or techniques described in this book, readers acknowledge and accept the inherent risks associated with physical activity and assume full responsibility for their own safety and well-being. The author of "Pickleball Power" shall not be held liable for any injuries, accidents, or damages that may occur as a result of utilizing the information provided in this book. Readers are encouraged to exercise caution, use proper equipment, and seek professional guidance when necessary to minimize the risk of injury.

Note from the Author

Welcome to the world of Pickleball Power, where the pursuit of health, fitness, and peak performance converge on the vibrant courts of this dynamic sport. In the following pages, you are about to embark on a transformative journey, one that promises to invigorate both your body and your spirit.

Pickleball, a game known for its blend of strategy, finesse, and athleticism, has captivated the hearts and minds of players of all ages and skill levels. It is a sport that epitomizes the joy of movement, camaraderie, and the thrill of competition, all wrapped up in the sound of paddles meeting a wiffle ball.

In *Pickleball Power: A Comprehensive Guide to Staying Healthy and Fit for Peak Performance,* you will find a wealth of knowledge, expertise, and inspiration. I am not only a passionate pickleball player but also a seasoned peak-performance and fitness professional with over twenty-seven years of experience who will provide you with the tools you need to excel in this exciting sport. I also understand that pickleball is more than just a game; it's a lifestyle, a way to stay active, and a pathway to wellness, which is why this book will help you play better for as long as you can.

This book goes beyond the rules and strategies of pickleball; it delves deep into the intricate relationship between your physical well-being and your on-court performance. You will discover a comprehensive approach to improving your strength, endurance, agility, and mental resilience, all tailored to the unique demands of pickleball. Whether you're a novice or a seasoned player, the insights within these pages will empower you to reach new heights in your game and in your overall health.

But this book is not only about training and technique. It is also a testament to the incredible sense of community that defines pickleball. It celebrates the friendships formed on the courts, the shared laughter, and the indomitable spirit of those who play this remarkable sport. It reminds us that pickleball is a vehicle for joy and well-being, a bridge that connects us across generations, backgrounds, and abilities.

As you delve into the pages of pickleball power, I encourage you to embrace the wisdom and guidance within and to carry it with you onto the courts. Whether you're seeking to elevate your pickleball game, enhance your fitness, or simply savor the delights of a healthy and active lifestyle, this book is your companion on that quest. It is a testament to the power of sport to transform lives, and it is a tribute to the vitality that pickleball brings to all who play it.

Get ready to unleash your potential, both on and off the court. Prepare to embark on a journey of Pickleball Power, where the pursuit of health and peak performance is a shared mission, and the possibilities are boundless.

Enjoy the game, embrace the challenge, and revel in Pickleball Power!

Sincerely,

Steve Jordan

Table of Contents

Introduction

The Growing Popularity of Pickleball

Pickleball, a paddle sport that combines elements of tennis, badminton, and table tennis, has experienced remarkable growth and made a significant impact worldwide in recent years. The game was invented in 1965 on Bainbridge Island, Washington, by Joel Pritchard, Bill Bell, and Barney McCallum.

The story goes that on a summer afternoon, Joel Pritchard, a congressman, and his friend Bill Bell returned to Pritchard's home after a game of golf to find their families bored and looking for something to do. They attempted to set up a game of badminton but couldn't find all the necessary equipment. Instead, they improvised using a wiffle ball, a lowered badminton net, and ping-pong paddles. The game that ensued was a combination of tennis, badminton, and ping-pong, played on a smaller court.

The name "pickleball" is said to have come from the Pritchard family's dog, Pickles, who would often chase after the ball during the game. However, Barney McCallum, one of the game's co-creators, claims that the name actually originates from the term "pickle boat" in crew, which refers to a boat that contains a mix of leftover oarsmen from other boats. The term was fitting because the game of pickleball combines elements from various sports.

Pickleball gained popularity quickly on Bainbridge Island and then spread to other parts of the United States and eventually internationally. It became especially popular among older adults due to its relatively low-impact nature compared to other racket sports like tennis, making it accessible to people of various ages and fitness levels.

Today, pickleball is played recreationally and competitively by millions of people worldwide, with organized tournaments, leagues, and clubs in many countries. Its growth continues as more people discover the fun and social aspects of the game. The growth of pickleball can be attributed to several key factors. First, its ease of learning and inclusivity has made it appealing to a diverse range of players, including seniors, children, and athletes of varying abilities. The sport's social and recreational nature has also made it a popular choice for those seeking physical activity and social interaction. Moreover, many communities and sports facilities have adapted their facilities to accommodate pickleball, helping to further its accessibility.

The emergence of professional pickleball has been nothing short of a remarkable journey in the world of sports. What was once a casual backyard game has evolved into a highly competitive and rapidly growing professional sport. Pickleball's ascent to professionalism can be attributed to a combination of factors, including its accessibility to people of all ages, a strong sense of community among players, and the desire for a new and exciting sport. As more and more athletes and enthusiasts embraced the game, tournaments began to grow in size and prestige. The formation of professional leagues and organizations, such as the Professional Pickleball Association (PPA) and the USA Pickleball

Association (USAPA), has further solidified the sport's professional status. Today, professional pickleball players are gaining recognition and sponsorship deals worth hundreds of thousands or even millions of dollars, and fans are eagerly tuning in to watch their favorite athletes compete in high-stakes matches. The emergence of pro pickleball has not only brought newfound attention to the sport but also inspired a new generation of players to aspire to reach the highest levels of competition in this exciting and fast-paced game.

Health and fitness are crucial in pickleball for several reasons:

Health and fitness play a crucial role in the game of pickleball, just as they do in any other sport. Pickleball is a fast-paced and physically demanding sport that requires agility, stamina, and strength. Maintaining good health and fitness levels is essential for several reasons.

1. **Endurance and stamina:** Pickleball can be a physically demanding sport, requiring players to move quickly, change directions, and maintain their energy levels throughout a game. Good fitness levels can help players maintain endurance and stamina.

2. **Injury prevention:** Being physically fit can reduce the risk of injuries, such as sprains or strains, which are common in pickleball due to sudden movements and quick changes in direction.

3. **Improved performance:** A strong and fit body can enhance your performance on the court, allowing you to react more quickly, maintain proper form, and execute shots effectively.

4. **Weight management:** Staying in good shape through fitness and exercise can help with weight management, which is important for overall health and can positively impact your agility and mobility on the pickleball court.

5. **Mental well-being:** Regular physical activity, including playing pickleball, is known to release endorphins and reduce stress. This can contribute to better mental health and focus on the game.

6. **Longevity:** Engaging in a sport like pickleball, which promotes physical activity, can help improve overall health and potentially extend one's lifespan.

In summary, optimal health and fitness play a vital role in enhancing one's performance, reducing the risk of injuries, and promoting overall well-being in pickleball, as in any other sport.

The Purpose of This Book

The main purpose of *Pickleball Power: A Comprehensive Guide to Staying Healthy and Fit for Peak Performance* is to promote and facilitate the overall well-being of pickleball players of all levels. This includes improving physical fitness, enhancing skills and techniques related to the sport, preventing injuries, and fostering a sense of community. This book aims to provide a holistic approach to pickleball, catering to the physical, mental, and social aspects of the game, ultimately helping players lead healthier and more fulfilling lives through their involvement in this fun and popular sport.

CHAPTER 1:

Understanding Pickleball

Rules and Basics

Knowing the rules and regulations of pickleball is crucial for several reasons, as it ensures a fair and enjoyable playing experience for all participants. First and foremost, understanding the rules promotes safety on the court for you and the other players. Pickleball involves rapid movement and precise shots, so adhering to the rules helps prevent accidents and injuries. For instance, players need to be aware of the no-volley zone (the *kitchen*) and foot faults to avoid stepping into these areas during play, reducing the risk of collisions.

Knowing the rules of the sport enhances the integrity of the game and contributes to the enjoyment of the game. The rules can be confusing at times—or at least they were for me when I first started to play, but the more you play, the more fundamental the rules become. Proper knowledge of scoring, serve rotations, and out-of-bounds calls helps maintain a level playing field and prevents disputes among players. Also, when players know the rules, they can strategize effectively, make informed decisions during play, and appreciate the game's nuances. It also encourages good sportsmanship and respect among competitors.

The Basics

Court: A pickleball court is a rectangular playing area used for the sport of pickleball, which is a paddle sport that combines elements of tennis, badminton, and table tennis. The court dimensions are similar to those of a doubles badminton court, measuring twenty feet wide and forty-four feet long for both singles and doubles play. The court is divided into different sections.

Baseline: The back boundary line of the court.

Sidelines: The two side boundary lines of the court.

Non-volley zone (NVZ): Also known as the *kitchen*, this is a seven-foot-deep area on each side of the net where players are not allowed to hit volleys. Players must let the ball bounce before hitting it if they are inside the NVZ.

Centerline: This line bisects the court perpendicular to the net, dividing it into two equal halves.

Service area: The service area is a rectangle measuring fifteen feet from the net to the baseline and extending to the sidelines.

Pickleball courts can be found both indoors and outdoors and are typically made of materials like concrete, asphalt, or wood. The surface of the court should be smooth and level to facilitate proper gameplay. The court layout and dimensions are standardized to ensure consistency and fairness in competition.

Pickleball Equipment

Pickleball paddle: A pickleball paddle is an essential piece of equipment used in the sport. It's similar to a tennis racket but smaller, typically measuring around eight to nine inches wide and fifteen to sixteen inches long. Pickleball paddles are made of various materials such as wood, graphite, composite, or a combination of materials. The core of the paddle can be made of materials like Nomex, aluminum, polymer, or foam.

Choosing the right pickleball paddle depends on factors like your playing style, skill level, and personal preferences. Paddles vary in weight, grip size, surface texture, and core material, so players often try out different paddles to find the one that suits them best. Some key considerations when selecting a pickleball paddle include the following:

- Weight: Paddle weights typically range from six to fourteen ounces. Lighter paddles offer more control and maneuverability, while heavier paddles provide more power. The ideal weight depends on your playing style and preferences.

- Grip size: Pickleball paddles come in various grip sizes to accommodate different hand sizes. A comfortable grip size ensures better control and prevents hand fatigue during extended play.

- Surface texture: Paddle surfaces may have a smooth finish or feature textured patterns like honeycomb or rough surfaces. Textured surfaces can add spin to the ball, while smooth surfaces offer better control and accuracy.

- Core material: The core material affects the paddle's feel, power, and control. Nomex cores are durable and provide a firm feel, while polymer cores offer a softer feel and more power. Foam cores are lightweight and absorb shock well.

- Edge guard: Some paddles feature an edge guard, which protects the paddle from damage during play and increases durability.

Ultimately, the best pickleball paddle for you depends on your playing style, preferences, and budget. It's a good idea to try out different paddles if possible to find the one that feels most comfortable and suits your game. Once you start playing pickleball, you will quickly realize how important your pickleball paddle is when working to improve your game. I tested close to a dozen different pickleball paddles in the past three years and found several brands worth mentioning.

I and other players are of the opinion that the best pickleball paddle for the most bang for the buck is the HEAD Radical Elite, due to its easy control and awesome price point of $70. My favorite overall is still the Onix Z5 graphite paddle, thanks to its combination of power and control for around $90. If you're someone who plays competitively and is looking for something more advanced, my recommendation is the Selkirk Halo Power XL, for its ability to deliver power and control.

The ball: The ball used in pickleball is similar to a wiffle ball, which is a plastic ball with holes. Pickleballs are specifically designed for the sport, being slightly larger than a standard wiffle ball. They are lightweight and have a certain amount of bounce, making them suitable for the fast-paced nature of pickleball. The color of pickleballs can vary, but they are often yellow, green, or white. My favorite ball, as seen on the cover of this book, is the Franklin X-40 for it's precise machine-drilled holes that ensure tight spin and a balanced flight pattern, all while still adhering to the USAPA specifications for tournament-approved balls.

The Pickleball Game

Singles and doubles: Pickleball can be played either in singles or doubles formats, each offering distinct challenges and strategies. In singles play, individuals cover the entire court, demanding agile movement and comprehensive court coverage. The strategy involves aiming shots to displace opponents and efficient court management. Singles players must master serve and return tactics to gain an early advantage. Conversely, doubles play divides the court between partners, emphasizing teamwork and communication. Coordinated efforts enable players to exploit gaps in opponents' defense, particularly at the net, where volleys and smashes are common. Doubles strategy often focuses on setting up partners for winning shots, with serves and returns tailored to maximize opportunities. Whether specializing in singles or doubles, players hone unique skill sets to excel in their preferred format.

Highlighted below are some of the key differences between singles and doubles play:

Singles Play

- **Court coverage:** In singles, players cover the entire court themselves, which means they need to be agile and have good court coverage.

- **Strategy:** Strategy in singles often involves trying to hit shots that pull your opponent out of position, as well as covering the court efficiently to defend against your opponent's shots.

- **Movement:** Singles requires a lot of movement, as players need to cover the court both horizontally and vertically. Quick footwork and good anticipation are essential.

- **Serve and return:** The serve and return are crucial in singles, as they set the tone for the point. A well-placed serve can put pressure on your opponent right from the start.

Doubles Play

- **Court coverage:** In doubles, players cover only half of the court, which means they can specialize in either the forehand or backhand side.

- **Teamwork:** Doubles play requires strong teamwork and communication between partners. Knowing when to cover for your partner and when to let them take a shot is key.

- **Strategy:** Strategy in doubles often involves setting up your partner for a winning shot, as well as trying to exploit the gaps between your opponents.

- **Net play:** Doubles play often involves more action at the net, with players trying to volley and smash shots to put pressure on their opponents.

- **Serve and return:** In doubles, the serve and return are still important, but players often use different strategies, such as serving to specific areas to exploit weaknesses in their opponents' positioning.

Ultimately, both formats offer unique challenges and enjoyment. Some players may prefer one over the other based on their playing style, fitness level, and social preferences. It's good to try both and see which one you enjoy more.

The Serve

In pickleball, the serve is a crucial element that sets the tone for each point. It's the starting shot that initiates the rally and offers players an opportunity to gain an advantage. The serve must be executed underhand and diagonally across the court to the opponent's service zone. With strict rules dictating the server's position behind the baseline and the ball's contact below waist level, precision and control are essential. A well-placed serve can limit the opponent's options, forcing them into a defensive position or setting up an offensive opportunity. Additionally, spin and speed variations can add complexity, making it challenging for the receiver to anticipate the ball's trajectory accurately. Mastering the serve is fundamental to success in pickleball, as it not only dictates the pace of the game but also influences strategy and player dynamics throughout the match.

Below are key points about the pickleball serve:

Service area: The serve must be made from behind the baseline, and it must land diagonally cross-court in the opponent's service court.

Service motion: The serve is typically an underhand motion. The server must keep one foot behind the baseline when serving and maintain contact with the ground until the ball is struck.

Double bounce rule: The serve must bounce once on the server's side and once on the receiver's side before being hit. After the two bounces, players can either volley the ball (hit it before it bounces) or let it bounce once before returning it.

Faults: If the serve doesn't land in the correct diagonal service court, hits the net and fails to go over, or goes out of bounds, it is considered a fault. Two consecutive faults result in a point for the opponent.

Foot faults: Stepping on or over the baseline or the center line during the serve is considered a foot fault.

Service rotation: In doubles play, both partners on a team will have the opportunity to serve, and the serve alternates between partners.

Server position: In doubles, the server can stand anywhere behind the baseline and within the sideline. However, they cannot step into the non-volley zone (often referred to as the kitchen) until after the ball has been struck.

Practice makes progress, especially when it comes to the serve, so don't be discouraged if it takes a while for you to find your rhythm. Practicing different serve types—such as the lob, drive, or slice—can provide you with a strategic advantage, allowing you to dictate the flow of the game from the very first shot.

Scoring

Scoring follows a straightforward system that adds a layer of excitement to the game. Matches are typically played to 11 points, although some variations may extend to 15 or 21 points. To win a point, a player or team must serve the ball and have it go unreturned by their opponents, either through a missed return or a fault. Unlike traditional tennis scoring, points can only be scored by the serving side. If the serving side wins a rally, they gain a point and continue to serve, alternating sides with each serve until the game is won. However, if the receiving side wins a rally, they don't score a point but instead gain the serve. This dynamic keeps the game fast-paced and ensures that both teams have an equal opportunity to score. Additionally, a two-point margin is typically required to win a game, meaning that if the score reaches 10–10, the game continues until one side leads by at least two points. Overall, pickleball scoring emphasizes skillful play and strategic serving, making each point a crucial moment in the match.

In/Out Rules

When serving, the ball must land in the diagonally opposite service court and clear the non-volley zone, also known as the kitchen, which extends seven feet from the net on both sides. During rallies, players must ensure the ball lands within the court boundaries. If the ball lands outside these lines or on the line itself, it is considered out. However, if there's doubt whether a ball is in or out, players may call for a judge's decision or mutually agree to replay the point. Fair play and sportsmanship are fundamental to the pickleball community, with players typically erring on the side of honesty when making calls.

Double Bounce Rule

The double bounce rule is a fundamental aspect that governs the game's flow and strategy. According to this rule, each team must allow the ball to bounce once on their side before they can return it. This ensures fairness and allows players ample opportunity to react to the opponent's shots. The double bounce rule encourages strategic placement of shots and rewards anticipation and positioning on the court. It adds an element of control and finesse to the game, as players must carefully judge when to let the ball bounce and when to make their move. By enforcing this rule, pickleball promotes a balanced and engaging playing experience for all involved, fostering skill development and tactical thinking among players of all levels.

Faults

Faults occur when players fail to adhere to the rules and regulations of the game. Common faults include stepping into the non-volley zone, also known as the *kitchen*, while hitting a volley, serving or returning the ball out of bounds, hitting the ball before it bounces once on each side of the net during the serve, and failing to let the ball bounce before volleying it. Additionally, faults can result from touching the net or its supports during play, deliberately distracting or obstructing opponents, or committing foot faults during the serve. These faults often lead to point deductions or loss of serve, emphasizing the importance of precise execution and adherence to the fundamental rules of pickleball.

Non-Volley Zone (Kitchen)

The kitchen in pickleball is a critical area on the court that spans seven feet from the net on both sides. It serves as a buffer zone where players cannot volley the ball directly out of the air. This rule promotes strategic placement and soft shots, enhancing the game's finesse and skill. The kitchen often becomes the focal point of intense rallies as players aim to maneuver their opponents into compromising positions while avoiding stepping into the forbidden zone. Mastering the dynamics of the kitchen requires precise footwork, a delicate touch, and keen anticipation, making it an integral part of the sport's tactical depth. It's where the battle for control and dominance is often decided, showcasing the essence of pickleball's competitive spirit and camaraderie.

Let Serves

Let serves add an element of unpredictability to the game, much like their counterparts in tennis. A let serve occurs when the ball hits the net during a serve but still lands within the correct serving court. Unlike tennis, where let serves are often replayed, in pickleball, let serves are generally considered valid, as long as they land in the proper service court. This means that a let serve can result in an unexpected bounce or trajectory, catching opponents off guard and potentially leading to an advantage for the serving team. Players must remain alert and ready to adapt to the ever-changing dynamics of the game, as let serves can introduce both challenges and opportunities during a match.

The Physical Demands of the Sport

The physical demands of pickleball primarily stem from the quick, dynamic movements required on the court. Players must exhibit good footwork, balance, and agility to cover the court efficiently and respond to fast-paced rallies. The game involves rapid changes in direction, sprinting to the net, and lateral movements, which demand cardiovascular endurance and leg strength. Hand-eye coordination and reflexes are crucial for precise shots and strategic play. While not as physically demanding as some high-intensity sports, pickleball still offers a great way to stay active and maintain a healthy lifestyle, making it an attractive option for individuals of various fitness levels. Pickleball is a relatively low-impact sport compared to many others, but it still has its physical demands. For peak performance, the following health and fitness attributes are essential:

Cardiovascular Endurance

The sport's rapid shifts in direction, explosive movements, and quick reflexes require efficient oxygen delivery to working muscles, prompting elevated heart rates and increased blood circulation. Players engage in continuous bursts of sprinting, lunging, and quick changes in direction, necessitating sustained cardiovascular endurance.

Muscular Strength

Muscular strength is crucial in executing powerful shots, making swift movements, and maintaining endurance throughout the game. Strong muscles, particularly in the arms, shoulders, and legs, enable players to deliver forceful serves, accurate volleys, and quick changes in direction on the court. A solid foundation of muscular strength not only enhances shot accuracy and power but also aids in injury prevention and overall performance consistency. Through targeted training and conditioning exercises as presented in this book, players can develop the muscular strength necessary to dominate rallies and outmaneuver opponents on the pickleball court.

Agility and Speed

Agility and speed are essential components for success on the court. Agile players possess the ability to swiftly change direction, react to opponents' shots, and cover the court effectively. Speed is crucial for reaching shots quickly and maintaining pressure on opponents. By honing agility through footwork drills and improving speed with targeted conditioning, players can enhance their overall performance, enabling them to anticipate plays, maneuver efficiently, and dominate rallies. In this fast-paced sport, mastering agility and speed can be the difference between victory and defeat.

Balance and Coordination

Balance and coordination are paramount in pickleball, where precise movement and control are key to success. Maintaining balance allows players to position themselves optimally for shots and swiftly adjust to changing game dynamics. Coordination, on the other hand, enables players to execute shots with accuracy and timing, whether it's a delicate drop shot or a powerful smash. Through practice drills that focus on footwork, body positioning, and hand-eye coordination, players can refine these skills, enhancing their ability to move fluidly around the court and execute shots with finesse. A solid foundation in balance and coordination not only improves performance but also reduces the risk of injury, ensuring that players can compete at their best.

Flexibility

Flexibility in pickleball offers a myriad of benefits to players of all levels. Primarily, it enhances agility and range of motion, allowing players to reach for shots more effectively and with reduced risk of injury. Flexibility aids in maintaining proper form throughout extended rallies, promoting better shot execution and consistency. And it fosters adaptability on the court, enabling players to adjust their positioning and shot selection to suit varying game situations and opponents' strategies. A flexible body enhances overall performance and enjoyment of the game, making it an indispensable asset.

Common Injuries in Pickleball

While it is generally considered a low-impact sport, there are still common injuries that players should be aware of. Unfortunately, frequent injuries in pickleball tend to be strains or sprains in the lower extremities, often resulting from sudden changes in direction or uneven court surfaces. Overuse injuries are also common and can occur due to repetitive playing without proper warm-up or cool-downs. It's important for pickleball enthusiasts to stay mindful of their physical well-being and take precautions to ensure a safe and enjoyable playing experience. Below are some of the common injuries that are occurring in pickleball players of all levels:

Sprains and strains: Injuries to ligaments and muscles can happen due to sudden movements, like quick changes in direction.

Tennis elbow (lateral epicondylitis): Overuse of the forearm muscles can lead to tennis elbow, causing pain and discomfort on the outer part of the elbow.

Rotator cuff injuries: Repetitive overhead shots can strain the shoulder's rotator cuff, leading to pain and limited mobility.

Knee injuries: Jumping, quick movements, and lateral shifts can put stress on the knee joints, leading to strains, sprains, or even tears.

Ankle injuries: Rolling or twisting the ankle is common when moving rapidly on the court.

Hamstring injuries: Sudden acceleration and deceleration can strain the hamstrings.

Achilles tendon injuries: Partial tears or complete rupture from too much stress on the ankles often necessitates surgical intervention and extensive rehabilitation to regain function and prevent long-term complications.

CHAPTER 2

The Mind-Body Connection

Mental Preparation and Focus

Mental preparation and focus are integral to success in pickleball, as they underpin various key aspects of the sport. The fast-paced and dynamic nature of pickleball demands unswerving concentration to track the ball's movement accurately, anticipate its trajectory, and make precise shot selections. Mental readiness also translates into quicker reaction times, facilitating the ability to reach and return shots effectively. Your focus plays a pivotal role in strategic decision-making, enabling players to formulate and adapt strategies on the fly, make split-second decisions, and choose the right shots and positioning.

Emotionally, mental preparation aids in managing the pressures and tensions of the game, enhancing resilience and the capacity to bounce back from setbacks. Maintaining consistency is another hallmark of successful pickleball players and is achieved through sustained mental focus throughout the match, ensuring steady and reliable play.

Confidence is closely intertwined with mental preparation because it boosts execution and performance. It is important to not self-judge and have a reflective mindset so you can analyze your performance and grow with each game, week, month, or year of play. Mental preparation and focus provide the foundation for a well-rounded and successful pickleball experience and ongoing development.

Techniques to Nurture Mental Resilience

Set clear goals: Clear goals provide direction, motivation, and a roadmap for progress. By clearly defining what you want to accomplish, you can better focus your efforts and resources toward reaching your desired outcome. You will be able to measure your progress, identify potential obstacles, and adjust your strategies accordingly.

Utilize visualization: By mentally rehearsing each shot, strategy, and movement on the court, you can sharpen your skills and develop a deeper understanding of the game. Visualizing successful serves, precise volleys, and strategic positioning can build confidence and focus, leading to improved performance during actual gameplay.

Stay in the present: Pickleball is not just a game. It's a meditation on the present moment. As the ball bounces across the court and the paddle swishes through the air, there's no room for past regrets or future worries. Each rally demands our full attention, and every shot is a testament to your focus and agility. In the heat of the match, time slows down, and all that matters is the next move. In these fleeting moments on the court, we find ourselves immersed in the pure joy of the game, anchored firmly in the present and flow.

Control your emotions: Mastering the art of controlling your emotions is as crucial as perfecting your technique. Whether you are facing a challenging opponent or dealing with a series of errors, maintaining composure is key to success. By staying focused and composed, you can make rational decisions, adapt your strategies effectively, and keep your performance at its peak. Emotions like frustration or anxiety can often cloud judgment and hinder gameplay. Through mindfulness techniques, deep breathing, and positive self-talk, you can regulate your emotions, stay present in the moment, and perform at your best.

Be adaptable: Being an adaptable player gives you the ability to react swiftly to your opponents moves, seamlessly transitioning between offensive and defensive plays as the game unfolds. Whether it's altering shot selection, changing positioning on the court, or adjusting to different playing styles, being adaptable in pickleball allows you to stay one step ahead and maintain control of the game.

Establish a routine: Establishing a pre-game routine helps you prepare physically and mentally, ensuring you are ready to play your best. Whether it's a specific warm-up routine, a ritual before serving, or a mental preparation routine to stay focused during intense rallies, having a set sequence of actions can help you maintain a rhythm and confidence throughout the game. A routine also provides a sense of comfort and familiarity, reducing anxiety and allowing you to focus solely on the game strategy and execution.

Do post-game analysis: This is a vital aspect of improving your skills and strategies on the court. After a match I recommend engaging in reflective discussions with your partner or opponents on your performance to help you identify strengths and pinpoint areas for improvement. Analyzing shot selection, movement patterns, communication with partners, and tactical decisions allows you to refine your game and adapt to different opponents in future matches.

It is important to keep in mind that mental preparation is a continuous process and takes a tremendous amount of discipline. Practice these aforementioned techniques regularly to enhance your mental resilience and performance.

The Role of Stress and Anxiety

The role of stress and anxiety in our lives can be a real health hazard and issue. I enjoy playing the game of pickleball because it allows me to relieve stress and anxiety from my personal and professional life. However, that stress and anxiety can be carried over onto the pickleball court if you are not aware of it or if you take the play too seriously. When overwhelmed by stress, you may experience decreased focus, leading to errors in judgment and technique. Anxiety can manifest as heightened tension in the muscles, impairing agility and coordination on the court. Stress may disrupt your sleep patterns, leaving you fatigued and less able to perform at your peak during matches. Long-term exposure to stress and anxiety in pickleball can contribute to burnout and diminished enjoyment of the sport, potentially leading to decreased participation over time.

Below, I've highlighted several areas that can give you an idea or indication that you may be bringing stress and anxiety to your pickleball play:

Performance: While some level of stress can enhance your performance, excessive anxiety will hinder it. You may experience decreased concentration, coordination, and decision-making during your matches.

Physical symptoms: Stress and anxiety can lead to physical symptoms like muscle tension, rapid heart rate, clammy hands, dry mouth, nervous ticks like biting nails, and even nausea.

Pre-competition nerves: Many people, including me, experience pre-competition nerves, known as "butterflies." Managing these feelings with some of the techniques mentioned above, like visualization, can help you use these "butterflies" to your advantage.

Choking: High levels of anxiety and stress can lead to "choking," where you will underperform in critical moments because you are often overthinking or you have a fear of failure.

Burnout: Prolonged stress and anxiety can contribute to burnout, leading to decreased motivation and overall well-being. To avoid burnout, it's essential to maintain a balanced approach to the sport. Listen to your body and recognize signs of fatigue or overexertion. Incorporate regular rest days into your training schedule to allow for proper recovery.

Inherent stress and anxiety are ubiquitous companions in the realm of all sports, including pickleball. The competitive nature of sport, combined with high stakes and intense scrutiny, can induce significant pressure. Develop resilience, mental fortitude, and effective coping strategies to navigate the tumultuous landscape of pickleball, harnessing the power of stress to propel yourself toward your goals rather than succumbing to its pressures. Remember to always have fun!

Strategies for Mental Toughness

Mental toughness in pickleball is a critical asset that can significantly enhance your performance and overall experience. It allows you to maintain focus and composure, even in the face of intense competition or challenging situations. This mental resilience helps you make better decisions, adapt to changing game conditions, and stay calm under pressure.

Mental toughness aids in the development of a positive and growth mindset. When you approach the game with strong mental resilience, you are more likely to approach each match with a winning attitude, believing in your ability to overcome obstacles and have fun. This confidence not only enhances your on-court performance but can also translate to other aspects of your life, promoting a healthy and confident self-image.

When you have mental toughness, you can foster better emotional control. When you can effectively manage your anxiety and frustration on the court, preventing yourself from making impulsive or rash decisions during a match, you'll find more enjoyment. This emotional regulation contributes to better sportsmanship and a more enjoyable experience for not just you, but everyone involved.

It is important to understand the difference between mental resilience and mental toughness as you approach these techniques below to help you create mental toughness. Mental toughness is about performing well in the face of stress and adversity, while mental resilience is about overcoming adversity and emerging stronger as a result.

Here are the ways to facilitate peak performance on the pickleball court:

Set clear goals: Define your objectives and break them down into smaller, more manageable steps. When you have well-defined objectives, you are better equipped to focus your energy and efforts, channeling them toward productive outcomes even in the face of challenges or setbacks.

Use positive self-talk: Replace negative thoughts with positive affirmations. Challenge self-doubt and maintain a growth mindset. Here are some examples of positive self-talk:

- I am capable and competent. I can handle whatever comes my way.

- I believe in myself and my abilities.

- I choose to focus on the present moment and let go of worries about the future.

- I am mentally tough. I have overcome challenges before, and I will overcome them again.

Visualize: Here are some visualization exercises:

- **Mental repetition of shots:** Close your eyes and mentally visualize yourself executing various shots in different game situations. Imagine yourself hitting a perfect serve, a powerful forehand drive, or a precise drop shot. Picture yourself moving fluidly around the court, anticipating your opponent's moves, and reacting with speed and accuracy.

- **Anticipation practice:** Visualize different game scenarios and anticipate your opponent's shots. Picture yourself reading your opponent's body language, predicting their shot selection, and positioning yourself accordingly to counter their moves effectively.

- **Strategic visualization:** Envision yourself using different strategies and tactics during a game. Picture yourself using lobs to push opponents back, executing dinks to control the net, or employing quick-reflex volleys to keep your opponents off balance. Visualize yourself adapting your strategy based on the score, your opponent's strengths and weaknesses, and the flow of the game.

Embrace failure: Failure isn't just accepted; it is an integral part of the journey toward mastery. Each missed shot, every imperfect serve, is a stepping stone toward growth and improvement. Embracing failure in pickleball means understanding that setbacks pave the way for learning, mental toughness, and, ultimately, success on the court.

Surround yourself with support: Build a strong support network of friends, family, or mentors who can provide encouragement and guidance when things go wrong, you are in a losing streak, you feel you need a pick-me-up.

Seek professional help: If you find yourself struggling with maintaining mental toughness while playing pickleball and feel that it's affecting your performance on the court, seeking professional help can be immensely beneficial. A trained mental toughness coach or sports psychologist can provide you with techniques to manage stress, stay focused, and maintain confidence during games.

Mental toughness is a skill that can be developed over time with practice and dedication. It's not about suppressing emotions, but rather learning how to channel them effectively to achieve your goals.

CHAPTER 3

Nutrition for Pickleball

Fueling Your Body

Nutrition plays a crucial role in pickleball, as it directly impacts an athlete's performance, endurance, and overall health on the court. Because of the fast-paced nature of pickleball and its physical demands of agility, quick reflexes, and sustained energy, proper nutrition is essential to meet these requirements and optimize your performance.

A balanced diet ensures that you have the necessary energy to maintain your stamina throughout a match. Carbohydrates are especially important, as they provide the primary source of energy for muscles. Protein is essential for muscle repair and growth, helping you recover from the physical strain of the game. Adequate hydration is also vital to prevent fatigue and cramping, as pickleball is often played in the heat, which can cause you to lose a significant amount of fluids through sweat.

Proper nutrition will also have a long-term impact on your overall health and well-being, reducing the risk of injuries and chronic conditions that any sport can cause but that are more common in the game of pickleball. Ingesting foods such as fruits, vegetables, and whole grains provides essential vitamins, minerals, and antioxidants, which can enhance recovery, reduce inflammation, and strengthen the immune system. Most professional sports teams have a sports nutritionist on staff because we now understand that a proper diet is a fundamental aspect of optimal performance in sports and life.

I have been working with clients for over twenty-five years helping them to tweak, alter, adapt, and reprogram their nutrition to help them with a variety of goals, including weight loss, improved sports performance, and aging well. Below are what I believe to be simple yet very effective ways to immediately begin to become more mindful of your nutrition for peak performance.

Pre-game nutrition: Aim for a balanced meal or snack that provides a combination of carbohydrates, protein, and healthy fats. Remember, carbohydrates fuel your muscles, so include foods like whole grains, fruits, and vegetables. Protein aids in muscle repair and recovery, so incorporate sources like lean meats, eggs, or plant-based options such as tofu or legumes. Healthy fats from sources like nuts, seeds, or avocados can provide sustained energy. Avoid heavy or greasy foods that could weigh you down, and aim to eat your pre-game meal or snack about one to three hours before playing to allow for digestion. Remember, everyone's nutritional needs may vary, so find what works best for you through experimentation, listening to your body's cues, and/or seeking professional help from a registered sports nutritionist. Visit www.zayacare.com for a sports nutritionist who can help you.

Simple and Nutritious Pre-Game Recipe:

Grilled Chicken and Quinoa Salad (serves 2 people)

Ingredients:

- ✓ 2 boneless, skinless chicken breasts

- ✓ 1 cup quinoa

- ✓ 2 cups water or chicken broth

- ✓ 1 red bell pepper, diced

- ✓ 1 cucumber, diced

- ✓ 1 cup cherry tomatoes, halved

- ✓ 2 cups mixed greens

- ✓ 1/4 cup chopped fresh cilantro

- ✓ Juice of 1 lemon

- ✓ 2 tablespoons olive oil

- ✓ Salt and pepper to taste

Instructions:

- ➢ Preheat your grill to medium-high heat.

- ➢ Season the chicken breasts with salt and pepper.

- ➢ Grill the chicken breasts for about 6–8 minutes per side, or until cooked through and no longer pink in the center.

Remove from the grill and let them rest for a few minutes before slicing.

> While the chicken is grilling, rinse the quinoa under cold water in a fine-mesh sieve. In a medium saucepan, combine the rinsed quinoa and water or chicken broth. Bring to a boil, then reduce the heat to low, cover, and simmer for about 15 minutes, or until the quinoa is cooked and the liquid is absorbed. Remove from heat and let it cool slightly.

> In a large mixing bowl, combine the cooked quinoa, diced bell pepper, cucumber, cherry tomatoes, mixed greens, and chopped cilantro.

> In a small bowl, whisk together the lemon juice and olive oil to make the dressing. Season with salt and pepper to taste.

> Add the sliced grilled chicken to the salad mixture.

> Drizzle the dressing over the salad and toss gently to coat everything evenly.

> Serve immediately, or refrigerate until ready to eat.

This recipe provides a good balance of carbohydrates, protein, and healthy fats to fuel your body before a game. Plus, it's packed with vitamins, minerals, and antioxidants from the vegetables and herbs.

Mindful snacking: Consuming nutrient-rich snacks such as fruits, nuts, or energy bars between matches helps replenish glycogen stores, providing a steady source of energy to sustain optimal performance. Snacking strategically can help you maintain focus and concentration by preventing dips in blood sugar levels, ultimately enhancing mental acuity and reaction time during intense rallies. Hydrating snacks like watermelon or coconut water aid in maintaining electrolyte balance, preventing fatigue, and ensuring endurance throughout the match. Mindful snacking during pickleball matches not only fuels the body but also sharpens the mind, enabling you to perform at your peak level and enjoy the game to the fullest.

Examples of Healthy Pre-Game Snacks

A healthy pre-game snack for optimal performance should provide a balance of carbohydrates, protein, and healthy fats to fuel your body and sustain energy levels. Here are some ideas:

- **Greek yogurt with berries and a sprinkle of granola:** Greek yogurt is rich in protein, while berries provide antioxidants and carbohydrates. Granola adds some healthy fats and additional carbohydrates for sustained energy.

- **Whole grain toast with almond butter and banana slices:** Whole grains provide complex carbohydrates, almond butter offers protein and healthy fats, and bananas supply potassium and easily digestible carbohydrates.

- **Trail mix with nuts, seeds, and dried fruit:** Nuts and seeds offer protein and healthy fats, while dried fruit provides quick energy from natural sugars. Just be mindful of portion sizes to avoid excess calories.

- **Hummus with veggie sticks:** Hummus is a good source of protein and healthy fats, while veggie sticks such as carrots, celery, and bell peppers provide carbohydrates and essential nutrients.

Five Quick Post-Game Snacks:

- **Protein smoothie:** This is an excellent choice for post-game recovery, as it provides a good balance of protein and carbohydrates. Plus, it's quick and easy to grab on the go.

- **Apple slices with almond butter:** Slice up an apple and dip the slices into almond butter for a satisfying combination of carbohydrates, healthy fats, and protein.

- **String cheese and whole-grain crackers:** Pair string cheese with whole-grain crackers for a quick and convenient snack that provides protein, calcium, and carbohydrates.

- **Greek yogurt with honey and berries:** Top Greek yogurt with a drizzle of honey and some fresh berries for a delicious and nutrient-rich snack that's packed with protein and antioxidants.

- **Turkey jerky:** Turkey jerky is a portable and protein-rich snack that can be easily eaten post-game to help replenish muscle stores and aid in recovery.

These snacks are not only quick to prepare but also provide the necessary nutrients to refuel your body after physical activity.

Post-game recovery: After an intense pickleball match, refueling your body with the right post-game recovery meal is essential for replenishing energy stores and aiding muscle repair. Optimal post-game meals for pickleball players should include a balance of carbohydrates to replenish glycogen stores, protein to support muscle recovery, and hydration to replace lost fluids. A nutritious option could be a turkey or chicken sandwich on whole grain bread with a side of fruit and a bottle of water or electrolyte-rich sports drink. Alternatively, a protein smoothie made with Greek yogurt, berries, and a scoop of protein powder can provide a quick and convenient recovery option. Whatever the choice, prioritizing nutrient-rich foods will help you recover faster and perform better in subsequent matches.

Simple and Nutritious Post-Game Recipe:

Here's a simple and nutritious post-game recipe that provides a good balance of carbohydrates, protein, and healthy fats to aid in recovery:

Turkey and Vegetable Salad with Ginger-Soy Dressing

Ingredients:

- ✓ 1 lb (450g) turkey breast, sliced thinly

- ✓ 4 cups mixed salad greens (such as spinach, arugula, and romaine lettuce)

- ✓ 2 cups mixed vegetables (such as bell peppers, broccoli, snap peas, carrots), thinly sliced

- ✓ 2 cloves garlic, minced

- ✓ 1 tablespoon ginger, grated

- ✓ 2 tablespoons low-sodium soy sauce

- ✓ 1 tablespoon hoisin sauce

- ✓ 1 tablespoon rice vinegar

- ✓ 1 tablespoon sesame oil

- ✓ 2 tablespoons olive oil

- ✓ Salt and pepper to taste

- ✓ Optional: sesame seeds and sliced green onions for garnish

Instructions:

- ➤ **Prepare the dressing:** In a small bowl, whisk together the minced garlic, grated ginger, soy sauce, hoisin sauce, rice vinegar, sesame oil, and olive oil until well combined. Set aside.

- ➤ **Stir-fry the turkey:** Heat one tablespoon of olive oil in a large skillet or wok over medium-high heat. Add the sliced turkey breast and stir-fry for 3–4 minutes until cooked through. Remove the turkey from the skillet and set aside.

- ➢ **Cook the vegetables:** In the same skillet, add the remaining tablespoon of olive oil. Add the mixed vegetables to the skillet and stir-fry for 4–5 minutes until they are tender-crisp.

- ➢ **Assemble the salad:** In a large salad bowl, combine the mixed salad greens, cooked turkey slices, and stir-fried vegetables.

- ➢ **Dress the salad:** Drizzle the prepared dressing over the salad and toss gently to coat everything evenly with the dressing.

- ➢ **Garnish and serve:** Garnish the salad with sesame seeds and sliced green onions if desired. Serve immediately.

This turkey and vegetable salad with ginger-soy dressing provides a refreshing and nutritious option for a post-game recovery meal after pickleball. It's packed with protein from the turkey, vitamins and minerals from the mixed greens and vegetables, and flavor from the delicious dressing. Enjoy your healthy salad!

Listen to your body: Listening to your body is paramount for maintaining overall well-being and optimal performance. Your body communicates its needs and limitations through various signals, such as pain, fatigue, hunger, and thirst. Ignoring these signals can lead to short-term or long-term physical and mental health issues. By paying attention to what your body is telling you, you can better understand its requirements and respond appropriately, whether it's getting adequate rest, nourishment, or hydration, or seeking medical attention when necessary.

Tuning into your body fosters self-awareness, empowers you to make healthier choices, and ultimately enhances your quality of life.

Nutrition is undeniably a deeply personal matter, as it intersects with individual preferences, cultural backgrounds, health conditions, and lifestyle choices. What works well for one person may not necessarily suit another. Personal dietary needs vary greatly, highlighting the importance of tailoring nutrition plans to meet individual requirements. Factors such as allergies, intolerances, ethical beliefs, and even taste preferences all play significant roles in shaping one's approach to food choices. Ultimately, achieving optimal nutrition involves understanding and honoring the unique needs and circumstances of each person, making it a highly personal journey toward health and well-being.

Hydration and Electrolyte Balance

Hydration and electrolyte balance are crucial in pickleball for several reasons. This fast-paced sport demands physical exertion and endurance, which can lead to significant sweating and fluid loss. Proper hydration ensures that you can maintain your energy levels, mental focus, and overall performance throughout a match. Pickleball, like other racket sports, requires precise muscle control and coordination, making electrolyte balance vital to prevent muscle cramps and maintain proper nerve function. Maintaining the right balance of electrolytes, such as sodium and potassium, aids in muscle function and helps prevent fatigue and injury. Therefore, staying adequately hydrated and maintaining electrolyte balance not only enhances your physical capabilities but also contributes to your safety and enjoyment on the pickleball court. Here are my top recommendations to maintain proper hydration and electrolyte balance:

Hydration: Adequate hydration regulates body temperature, enhances muscle function, and sustains cognitive sharpness, all crucial for sustained gameplay. Without proper hydration, players risk fatigue, cramping, and diminished focus, hindering their ability to execute precise shots and make strategic decisions. Whether in casual matches or competitive tournaments, prioritizing hydration empowers pickleball enthusiasts to maximize their potential, prolong their endurance, and enjoy the game to its fullest. Current sports nutrition science recommends that adults should drink 6–12 ounces /.18 –.35 liters of water per 20 minutes of play and teens 13–18 ounces /.35–.38 liters per 20 minutes of play. I also recommend drinking half your body weight in ounces of water per day. For example, If you weigh 150 lbs. /68 kilos, you would consume 75 ounces/2.2 liters of water per day.

Electrolytes: It is recommended by sports nutritionists that players should consume electrolyte-rich beverages, such as sports drinks or coconut water, before, during, and after play to replenish sodium, potassium, magnesium, and calcium lost through sweat, especially in hot conditions indoor or outdoor. Also, you want to incorporate foods rich in electrolytes, such as bananas, oranges, and leafy greens, into your pre-game meals to help support your electrolyte balance.

Monitor sweat loss: Monitoring sweat loss is essential to play optimally, especially in hot and humid conditions. To effectively monitor sweat loss, you can employ several methods. One approach is to weigh yourself before and after your play, accounting for fluid intake during your matches. Each pound lost typically represents approximately 16 ounces of fluid loss. Another method involves observing the color of urine; darker urine indicates dehydration. Using these techniques collectively can help you maintain proper hydration levels and optimize performance during play or practice.

Avoid overhydration: Overhydration can be just as detrimental as dehydration. When you consume excessive amounts of fluids, you risk diluting the body's electrolyte balance, leading to a condition called *hyponatremia*. This imbalance can impair muscle function and cognitive performance and even pose serious health risks. Therefore, it's essential for you to find that balance in your fluid intake by using any or all of the methods above.

CHAPTER 4:

Physical Conditioning

Functional Strength Training

Foundational strength training plays a crucial role in enhancing your performance in pickleball because pickleball demands a combination of agility, speed, and power, making it essential for you to develop your lower body, upper body, and core strength. A strong and well-conditioned body and core not only helps you maintain your stamina throughout a match, but also enables you to execute powerful shots, quick lateral movements, and effective net play. I recommend all pickleball players of all levels incorporate a functional strength training program that aids in preventing injuries and improves your coordination, reaction time, and balance by strengthening the muscles, ligaments, and tendons that stabilize joints required for the sport's dynamic movements from the inside out. Having functional strength can contribute to improved shot control and the ability to generate more force in serves and volleys, ultimately giving you a competitive edge. For these reason and so many more, functional strength training should be a vital component of all pickleball players' preparation, leading to improved performance, endurance, and overall enjoyment of the game at any age.

It is impossible to prescribe a functional strength program that would adequately address everyone's needs and wants. Therefore, here is a general overview of what should be included in your functional strength training program that either you or a private strength coach can program for you. I am also available for consults virtually and will have a stream of exercise programs available on the website: www.pickleballpowerbook.com.

Compound exercises: Compound movements are essential in pickleball, combining multiple muscle groups to execute powerful shots and swift movements on the court. These movements, such as the serve, forehand, and backhand strokes, require coordinated efforts from the legs, core, and upper body. Engaging in compound movements like squats, lunges, deadlifts, push-ups, overhead presses, and rows not only enhances functional strength but also improves overall performance and endurance during intense gameplay. By incorporating these dynamic movements into your fitness routine three times per week, you will effectively control the pace of the game and outmaneuver opponents with precision and finesse.

Core strength: Core strength is essential in pickleball, as it serves as the foundation for power, stability, and agility on the court. A strong core enables you to generate explosive movements for shots, swiftly change direction to reach balls, and maintain balance during quick-paced rallies. Whether it's executing powerful serves, driving precise shots, or swiftly maneuvering across the court, a strong core enhances your performance and prevents injuries. With a strong core, you'll be able to optimize your overall game, ensuring you are agile, stable, and capable of executing your shots with precision and power.

Plyometrics: Plyometric training enhances agility, power, and explosive movements crucial for competitive success. By incorporating plyometric exercises like jumps, hops, and bounds into your fitness program, you can improve your ability to react swiftly, explode into shots, and recover quickly during rallies. The dynamic nature of pickleball demands rapid changes in direction and sudden bursts of speed, all of which are honed through plyometric training. Plyometrics help fortify muscles, joints, and tendons, reducing the risk of injuries common in a fast-paced sport like pickleball. It is essential to integrate plyometric exercises into training regimens to significantly elevate your performance on the court.

Sport-specific movements: To enhance performance on the court, incorporating sports-specific exercises will help you play with grace and ease. Focus on drills that emphasize quick lateral movements to improve agility and footwork, as well as exercises targeting shoulder and core strength for powerful shots and stability during gameplay. Some of my favorite drills to help my clients play better pickleball are the side shuffle drill, figure eight drill, agility ladder, cone slalom drill, and ball reaction drills.

Balance training: Balance training is, in my opinion, the secret sauce for all sports, including pickleball, as it enhances your stability, agility, and overall performance on the court. Given the rapid shifts in direction and the quick-paced nature of the game, maintaining balance becomes a critical factor in executing shots effectively while reducing the risk of injury. A well-developed sense of balance enables you to move swiftly, react promptly to your opponent's shots, and maintain optimal positioning throughout the match. Incorporating balance exercises into your training routine and daily life will not only improve physical coordination but also enhance your mental focus, allowing you to make split-second decisions with confidence. Single-leg balance for 1 minute on each leg, BOSU ball two-leg or single-leg balance for 1 minute, balance board two-leg 1-minute balance, and single-leg net volley are great exercises to improve your balance. Visit www.pickleballpowerbook.com/balancetraining for more balance exercise examples that will include programming.

Recovery: Recovery plays a crucial role in maintaining peak performance and preventing injuries. It's during recovery periods that the body repairs and strengthens muscles, replenishes energy stores, and restores balance. In a fast-paced game like pickleball, where quick movements and agility are key, effective recovery strategies ensure you can sustain your intensity throughout matches. Adequate rest, hydration, nutrition, and stretching are vital components of a comprehensive recovery plan, helping you bounce back faster and perform at your best on the court. Ignoring recovery can lead to fatigue, decreased performance, and increased risk of injury, underscoring the importance of prioritizing rest and recovery alongside training and gameplay.

Cardiovascular Fitness

Cardiovascular training in pickleball offers a wide range of benefits to players of all skill levels. When played well, pickleball is a fast-paced sport that demands agility, quick reactions, and sustained bursts of energy, making cardiovascular fitness a key component for success and remarkable improvements in performance. Regular cardio workouts will improve your endurance, allowing you to maintain high energy levels throughout a match and reducing the risk of fatigue. Enhanced cardiovascular health also promotes better circulation and oxygen delivery to muscles, which will lead to improved performance and quicker recovery between points.

Focusing on a cardiovascular training program should be a part of pickleball preparation to not only boost overall physical fitness, but to lower the risk of heart disease and contribute to a healthier and more active lifestyle. So whether you're a casual player or a competitive enthusiast, incorporating cardiovascular training into your pickleball routine 2–4 times per week for 20–30 minutes can help you elevate your game and enjoy the sport to the fullest.

Below are just a few examples of cardiovascular exercises that I recommend to my pickleball clients, and there are many other activities you can explore to keep your heart healthy and improve your overall fitness level. It's essential to choose activities that you enjoy and can incorporate into your regular exercise routine for long-term adherence.

Running: Running is a highly effective cardio exercise that can be done outdoors or on a treadmill. It helps to improve endurance, burn calories, and strengthen the heart.

Cycling: Cycling, whether it's stationary or outdoors, is a great low-impact cardio workout. It strengthens the leg muscles and improves cardiovascular health.

Swimming: Swimming is a full-body workout that engages all major muscle groups. It's gentle on the joints and an excellent option for those with joint pain or injuries.

Jumping rope: Jumping rope is a simple yet effective cardio exercise that can be done almost anywhere. It improves coordination, agility, and cardiovascular health.

Brisk walking: Walking at a brisk pace is an accessible and low-impact cardio exercise suitable for all fitness levels. You can incorporate it into your daily routine by walking outdoors or on a treadmill.

High-intensity interval training (HIIT): HIIT involves alternating between short bursts of intense exercise and brief rest periods. It's a time-efficient way to improve cardiovascular fitness and burn calories.

Dancing: Dancing is a fun and enjoyable way to get your heart rate up while improving coordination and flexibility. You can try various dance styles, such as salsa, hip-hop, or Zumba.

Rowing: Rowing is a full-body workout that engages the arms, legs, and core muscles. It provides an effective cardiovascular workout while also strengthening muscles and improving posture.

Stair climbing: Climbing stairs is a simple yet effective cardio exercise that targets the lower body muscles and elevates the heart rate. You can use stairs at home or work or find a stair-climbing machine at the gym.

Kickboxing: Kickboxing combines cardio with strength training, making it a high-intensity workout that burns calories and improves cardiovascular health. It also helps to improve balance and coordination.

Flexibility and Mobility

Flexibility and mobility play crucial roles in enhancing peak performance in pickleball. These attributes provide a range of benefits for players of all skill levels. Flexibility in the joints and muscles allows you to execute a broader spectrum of shots, including those requiring a wide range of motion and agility. This versatility is particularly advantageous in pickleball, where quick reflexes and rapid changes in direction are essential for success.

Mobility ensures that you can effortlessly cover the entire court, both in singles and doubles play. Being able to move swiftly and transition from one area to another enhances your defensive and offensive capabilities, as you can reach more balls and maintain better court positioning. Having both flexibility and mobility helps to reduce the risk of injury, as it ensures you execute movements with proper form, minimizing the strain on joints and muscles. Overall, these attributes are fundamental in achieving success in pickleball, as they enable you to maintain a competitive edge, stay agile on the court, and enjoy the sport with reduced risk of injury. To improve your flexibility and mobility for peak performance, I strongly recommend incorporating this program daily or, at the very least, on the days you play.

Here are some great flexibility exercises you can incorporate into your program today, or visit www.pickleballpowerbook.com/flexibilitytraining for more flexibility exercise examples.

Leg swings: Stand next to a wall or sturdy object for support. Swing one leg forward and backward, then side to side in a controlled motion. Repeat for 10–15 swings on each leg.

Arm circles: Stand with your feet shoulder-width apart. Extend your arms out to the sides at shoulder height. Make small circles forward for 10–15 repetitions, then reverse the direction for another 10–15 repetitions.

Hip flexor stretch: Stand with feet hip-width apart. Take a step back with your right leg, keeping it straight. Bend your left knee and lean forward slightly, feeling a stretch in the front of your right hip. Hold for 20–30 seconds, then switch legs.

Hamstring stretch: Sit on the floor with one leg extended straight out in front of you and the other leg bent with the foot flat against the inner thigh of the extended leg. Lean forward from your hips, reaching toward your toes. Hold for 20–30 seconds, then switch legs.

Calf stretch: Stand facing a wall with your hands against it at shoulder height. Step one foot back, keeping it straight, and press your heel into the ground. Lean forward slightly to feel a stretch in the calf of the back leg. Hold for 20–30 seconds, then switch legs.

Torso twists: Stand with feet shoulder-width apart. Extend your arms out to the sides at shoulder height. Twist your torso to the right, bringing your left hand across your body to touch your right hand; then twist to the left, bringing your right hand across your body to touch your left hand. Repeat for 10–15 twists on each side.

Shoulder stretch: Stand or sit tall. Bring one arm across your body at chest height, using the opposite hand to gently press the arm toward your chest until you feel a stretch in the shoulder. Hold for 20–30 seconds, then switch arms.

Neck stretch: Sit or stand tall. Tilt your head to the right, bringing your right ear toward your right shoulder until you feel a stretch along the left side of your neck. Hold for 20–30 seconds, and then switch sides.

CHAPTER 5:

Injury Prevention

Injury prevention is paramount for all pickleball players to maintain physical health, have longevity in the sport, and enhance optimal performance on the court. Despite its reputation as a low-impact activity, pickleball still carries inherent risks, especially for players who engage in frequent and intense matches. Understanding the importance of injury prevention not only safeguards you from immediate harm but also ensures you can continue enjoying the game for years to come.

If you are physically fit and free from injury, you can move more efficiently, react quicker, and execute shots with greater precision. By incorporating functional strength training, flexibility exercises, and proper warm-up routines into your exercise regimen, you can improve your agility, endurance, and overall athleticism. This not only reduces the likelihood of acute injuries during play but also helps prevent overuse injuries that can develop over time.

Injury prevention fosters a culture of safety within the pickleball community. By prioritizing proper technique and adhering to safety guidelines, you'll help set a positive example for newcomers and fellow enthusiasts. This proactive approach not only reduces the risk of accidents and injuries during matches but also promotes a sense of camaraderie and respect among players. Club owners or coaches who are promoting injury prevention initiatives, such as workshops and educational resources, can empower players to take ownership of their health and well-being, ultimately creating a more inclusive and sustainable pickleball environment.

In addition to enhancing performance and fostering a culture of safety, injury prevention plays a crucial role in promoting overall health and well-being. It should not be taken for granted or understated that regular physical activity, such as playing pickleball, offers numerous health benefits, including improved cardiovascular health, weight management, and stress reduction. However, these benefits can be compromised if players are sidelined by injuries. Therefore, by adopting a comprehensive approach to injury prevention, which includes proper nutrition, hydration, and recovery strategies, pickleball players can maximize their potential both on and off the court. Ultimately, prioritizing injury prevention not only safeguards your health but also ensures you can continue enjoying the thrill of pickleball consistently and for a long time.

Warm-Up and Cool-Down Techniques

Warm-Up Techniques

Cardiovascular Warm-Up: Incorporating a cardiovascular warm-up routine is essential to prepare the body for any kind of physical activity. A brisk jog around the court or a few minutes of jumping jacks can elevate the heart rate and increase blood flow to the muscles, priming them for optimal performance. By dedicating just a few minutes to a cardiovascular warm-up, you can enhance your agility, endurance, and overall enjoyment of the game.

Dynamic flexibility: Dynamic flexibility allows you to swiftly maneuver around the court, reach for shots, and maintain agility throughout the game. Unlike static flexibility, which focuses on holding positions, dynamic flexibility involves fluid movements that mimic those encountered during gameplay. Incorporating dynamic stretches such as leg swings, arm circles, and torso twists into pre-match warm-ups enhances muscle elasticity and range of motion, enabling you to react quickly to unpredictable shots and maintain peak performance during intense rallies. By prioritizing dynamic flexibility, you'll be able to improve your agility, reduce the risk of injury, and elevate your overall on-court prowess. Examples of dynamic stretches are leg swings, arm circles, torso twists, high knees, and butt kicks. Visit www.pickleballpowerbook.com/dynamicflexibility for more exercises.

Pickleball-specific drills: Specific pickleball drills play a pivotal role in enhancing your skills and readiness before stepping onto the court. They provide focused practice on fundamental aspects such as control, accuracy, footwork, and strategy, which are essential for success during gameplay. By engaging in drills tailored to different aspects of the game, you can refine your techniques, build muscle memory, and develop the necessary agility and coordination required for competitive play. These specific drills also offer an opportunity for you to identify weaknesses and areas needing improvement, allowing you to target those areas effectively and continually evolve. Here are some great pickleball-specific drills you can work on:

Dinking Drill:

Purpose: To improve control and touch for soft shots at the net.

Setup: Two players on each side of the net, close to the kitchen line. Instructions: Rally back and forth, keeping the ball low and controlled. Focus on using the wrist to angle the paddle for placement rather than power.

Third Shot Drop Drill:

Purpose: To master the third shot, which is crucial for regaining control of the net.

Setup: One player at the net, one player at the baseline.

Instructions: The player at the baseline hits a deep serve, and the net player responds with a soft, controlled shot (the third shot drop) aimed at landing just beyond the net.

Volley Drill:

Purpose: To improve volleying skills and reaction time at the net.

Setup: Two players at the net on opposite sides.

Instructions: Players volley back and forth, focusing on keeping the ball low and controlled. Vary the pace and angle of shots to challenge each other.

Cool-Down Techniques:

Cool-down exercises in pickleball are essential for aiding the body's transition from intense activity to a state of rest. As with any physical activity, pickleball engages muscles, increases heart rate, and elevates body temperature. Cool-down exercises will help you gradually decrease your heart rate, prevent muscle stiffness, and reduce the risk of injury by promoting blood flow and removing lactic acid buildup. Additionally, they will help you to mentally unwind and reflect on your game performance. Incorporating cool-down exercises into a pickleball routine not only enhances physical recovery but also contributes to your overall well-being, ensuring you can consistently enjoy the sport while minimizing the chances of injury. The following are some of my favorite pickleball cool-down techniques. Visit www.pickleballpowerbook.com/cooldown for more.

Static stretches: Incorporating static stretches into your post-pickleball routine offers numerous benefits for your body and overall performance. These stretches help alleviate muscle tension and soreness by gradually lengthening and relaxing the muscles, promoting better blood circulation and nutrient delivery to the tissues. By cooling down with static stretches, you can improve flexibility and joint range of motion, and reduce the risk of injury by allowing your body to return to its resting state gradually.

Hamstring stretch: Sit on the ground with one leg extended straight in front of you and the other bent, with the sole of the foot against the inner thigh. Reach forward and gently grasp the toes or ankle of the extended leg, keeping the back straight. Hold the stretch for 20–30 seconds and then switch legs.

Quadriceps stretch: Stand tall and grab one ankle behind you, pulling it toward your glutes. Keep your knees close together and your torso upright. Hold the stretch for 20–30 seconds and then switch legs.

Calf stretch: Stand facing a wall with one foot forward and the other back, both feet pointing forward. Lean forward, keeping the back heel on the ground until you feel a stretch in the calf of the back leg. Hold for 20–30 seconds and then switch legs.

Shoulder stretch: Bring one arm across your body, holding it at the elbow with your opposite hand. Gently pull the arm toward your chest until you feel a stretch in the shoulder. Hold for 20–30 seconds and then switch arms.

Foam rolling: Foam rolling during cool down offers a myriad of benefits. By engaging in foam rolling post pickleball matches, you can effectively alleviate muscle tension and soreness accumulated during your play. This self-myofascial release technique promotes blood circulation, aiding in the removal of metabolic waste products from muscles and reducing the risk of delayed onset muscle soreness (DOMS). Foam rolling also enhances flexibility and range of motion by breaking down adhesions or knots in the muscle fascia, thus improving overall athletic performance and preventing injuries. Incorporating foam rolling into a cool-down routine not only enhances recovery but also promotes relaxation, leaving individuals feeling rejuvenated and ready for their next training session.

Visit www.pickleballpowerbook.com/foamrolling for foam rolling programs and instruction.

Breathing exercises: After a vigorous game of pickleball, taking the time to engage in controlled breathing exercises offers numerous benefits for a thorough cooldown. Deep, intentional breaths help to regulate heart rate and bring it back to a resting state, promoting relaxation and reducing muscle tension. Oxygenating the body through focused breathing aids in clearing out any accumulated lactic acid and metabolic waste, which can alleviate soreness and promote quicker recovery. Mindful breathing fosters mental clarity and concentration, allowing you to reflect on your performance and set intentions for future play. Incorporating breathing techniques into a post-pickleball cooldown routine not only enhances physical recovery but also promotes overall well-being and mindfulness. Visit www.pickleballpowerbook.com/breathingexercises for a breathing program and instruction.

The Importance of Rest and Recovery

Rest and recovery are essential for peak pickleball performance. As mentioned several times in this book, pickleball is fast-paced and is a physically demanding sport that places significant strain on the body. The importance of rest and recovery cannot be overstated, as it directly impacts optimal performance, well-being, and overall longevity in the game.

When you engage in pickleball, your body undergoes various physical stresses, such as sprinting, pivoting, and intense rallies. These activities can lead to muscle fatigue, micro-injuries, and mental fatigue. Rest and recovery provide the much-needed opportunity for the body to repair and rebuild, which is crucial for maintaining optimal performance and preventing overuse injuries.

Taking breaks between games or training sessions allows the body to replenish energy stores, reduces the risk of injuries, and improves overall fitness levels. Adequate rest also plays a vital role in maintaining mental focus and enthusiasm for the sport, helping you remain motivated and engaged.

Proper rest and recovery strategies, including stretching, hydration, and nutrition, are fundamental for enhancing your endurance and resilience. By prioritizing rest and recovery, you can maximize your potential on the court and enjoy a longer, healthier, and more fulfilling pickleball journey. I would consider rest and recovery as the unsung heroes that support all players in their pursuit of excellence.

Rest and Recovery Examples

Active recovery days: Active recovery days are crucial components of any fitness and pickleball schedule, offering a deliberate break from intense workouts while still promoting movement and circulation. These days are characterized by low-impact exercises such as walking, swimming, or gentle yoga, which help to alleviate muscle soreness, enhance flexibility, and facilitate recovery. By engaging in light physical activity, you can maintain momentum in your health and fitness journey without overtaxing your body, ultimately promoting overall well-being and long-term sustainability to play pickleball at optimal levels.

Massage therapy: Massage therapy offers numerous benefits to aid in recovery after intense pickleball matches and play. It helps to improve blood circulation, which promotes the delivery of oxygen and nutrients to damaged tissues, speeding up the healing process. Massage also reduces muscle tension and stiffness by loosening knots and releasing built-up lactic acid, which can alleviate soreness and improve flexibility. It also stimulates the lymphatic system, facilitating the removal of toxins and waste products from the body, further enhancing the recovery process. Beyond the physical benefits, massage also promotes relaxation and reduces stress, which can contribute to overall well-being and faster recovery. Incorporating massage therapy into a recovery regimen can significantly enhance your body's ability to rest and recover better.

Hydration and nutrition: As stated earlier in chapter 3, staying properly hydrated before, during, and after pickleball sessions is essential and also very important to aid in optimal recovery. Replenishing electrolytes lost through sweating and feeding your muscles with protein to rebuild and restore is also a key factor. If you don't understand anything else about nutrition, you can use this simple rule of thumb: prioritize nutrient-rich foods like leafy greens, fish, chicken, lean meat, avocados, sweet potatoes, eggs, and yogurt.

Sleep: Sleep is not merely a luxury. It's a fundamental pillar of optimal performance. It serves as the body's crucial restoration period, essential for cognitive function, emotional well-being, and physical health. During sleep, the brain consolidates memories, processes information, and rejuvenates neural pathways, fostering creativity, problem-solving abilities, and learning retention. Sufficient sleep bolsters immune function, regulates metabolism, and promotes overall physical recovery. Without it, you may experience diminished focus, heightened stress levels, and decreased productivity. Prioritizing quality sleep is paramount for achieving peak performance in every aspect of life, including pickleball. Aim for seven to nine hours of quality sleep each night.

Rest days: Rest days are indispensable for achieving optimal performance in your health and fitness. Rest days allow the body and mind crucial time to recover, repair, and rejuvenate. Physically, rest days prevent overtraining, reducing the risk of injury and muscle fatigue while promoting muscle growth and repair. Mentally, they offer a chance to unwind, recharge, and maintain focus and motivation. Ignoring rest can lead to burnout, decreased performance, and increased susceptibility to illness or injury on or off the pickleball court. By incorporating rest days into your routine, you can ensure long-term success, sustainability, and overall well-being.

Contrast water therapy: Contrast water therapy is a technique alternating between hot and cold water immersion and holds significant importance in your rest and recovery. The stark contrast in temperatures stimulates circulation, promoting blood flow and lymphatic drainage, which aids in reducing inflammation and expediting recovery from injuries.Contrast water therapy helps in alleviating muscle soreness, enhancing joint mobility, and promoting relaxation. Its simplicity and effectiveness make it a valuable adjunct to physical therapy regimes, enabling you to recover faster and maintain optimal performance levels.

Low-intensity cross-training: Low-intensity cross-training plays a pivotal role in enhancing optimal performance by offering a variety of benefits to athletes and fitness enthusiasts. Incorporating activities such as swimming, cycling, or yoga alongside regular training routines and playing pickleball helps you to reduce the risk of overuse injuries by providing active recovery periods. It also promotes muscular balance and prevents burnout by engaging different muscle groups and movement patterns than those use in when playing pickleball. This type of training aids in improving cardiovascular endurance and overall fitness levels while allowing for adequate rest and recovery from high-intensity workouts. Low-intensity cross-training also fosters mental rejuvenation, reducing stress and enhancing focus, thus contributing to long-term performance gains.

Listen to your body: Ignoring the signals of fatigue or pushing through pain can lead to burnout, injury, and decreased performance. Tuning in to your body will provide subtle cues, such as fatigue, soreness, and decreased energy levels. Prioritizing rest and recovery is fundamental to achieving your peak potential.

Injury Rehabilitation

In the event of an injury sustained from playing pickleball, it is crucial to prioritize your well-being and take appropriate steps for a swift and safe recovery. First, assess the severity of the injury. If it's a minor issue like a sprain, strain, or a small scrape, it's advisable to stop playing immediately to prevent further damage. Rest, ice, compression, and elevation (RICE) can be helpful in managing minor injuries. Apply ice to reduce swelling, compress the injured area, and keep it elevated to minimize inflammation.

For more serious injuries, such as a fracture, head injury, or muscle tear, it's essential to seek immediate medical attention. Do not attempt to continue playing, and call for professional help or go to the nearest medical facility as soon as possible.

Regardless of the injury's severity, it's crucial to listen to your body and not push through the pain. It is imperative that you rest and allow your body time to heal. Once you have received medical advice or treatment, follow the prescribed rehabilitation and recovery plan. Always remember to warm up before playing and wear appropriate protective gear like knee, elbow pads, and eye protection, if needed, to reduce the risk of injury during your pickleball matches. Safety should always be a top priority.

Here are some general steps to consider if you're dealing with a pickleball-related injury:

Diagnosis: First, get a proper diagnosis from a medical professional. This may involve X-rays, MRI scans, or other tests to determine the extent and nature of your injury.

Rest: In many cases, rest is crucial to allow the injured area to heal. Follow your healthcare provider's advice on when and how to rest.

Physical therapy: If recommended, attend physical therapy sessions. A trained therapist can guide you through exercises and stretches to regain strength and flexibility.

Pain management: Use pain management techniques such as ice, heat, or over-the-counter pain relievers as advised by your healthcare provider.

Gradual return: When cleared by your healthcare provider, gradually reintroduce pickleball into your routine. Start with low-intensity practice and slowly increase the intensity.

Proper technique: Ensure your playing technique is sound to prevent future injuries. Consider getting coaching or guidance if needed.

Strength and conditioning: Work on strengthening and conditioning the muscles and joints related to pickleball to reduce the risk of reinjury.

Nutrition and hydration: A balanced diet and proper hydration play a significant role in the healing process and overall well-being.

CHAPTER 6:

Pickleball-Specific Training

Drills and Practice Routines

Drills and practice routines play a pivotal role in the development and success of pickleball players at all skill levels. Pickleball requires a unique set of skills, including precision, agility, and strategic thinking that is unique to this sport. Regular drills and practice sessions will not only help you refine your techniques but also build essential muscle memory that will improve your overall game. Whether it's perfecting the art of the serve, mastering dink shots at the net, or honing defensive maneuvers, these structured practice sessions will allow you to isolate specific aspects of your game for targeted improvement.

Consistent practice not only increases physical endurance but also sharpens mental acuity, as players learn to anticipate opponents' moves and formulate winning strategies. With a little bit of discipline and focus, you can elevate your game, compete at a higher level sooner, and derive greater enjoyment from the sport. Like any sport where precision and strategy are paramount, drills and practice routines are the foundation upon which you will improve your skills to achieve your personal goals. Here are some fun and challenging drills that are sure to improve your game and play:

Footwork Drill:

Purpose: To enhance agility and movement on the court.

Setup: Set up cones or markers to create a footwork grid on the court.

Instructions: Players move around the grid, practicing different footwork patterns such as side shuffles, crossover steps, and split steps. Emphasize quick movements and proper positioning.

Serve and Return Drill:

Purpose: To work on serving accuracy and returning serves effectively.

Setup: Two players on each side of the net.

Instructions: One player serves while the other focuses on returning the serve with placement and control. Alternate roles after a set number of serves.

Dinking Drill:

Purpose: The purpose of the dinking drill is to improve your ability to maintain a soft touch on the ball and to control its placement over the net, which is crucial for maintaining rallies and setting up winning shots.

Setup: Players stand on opposite sides of the net at the kitchen line (non-volley zone line), facing each other.

Instructions: One player begins by softly hitting (dinking) the ball over the net to the other player, aiming to land the ball in the non-volley zone (kitchen) on the other side. The receiving player then hits the ball back with a soft touch, aiming to keep it low and controlled. Players continue to exchange soft shots back and forth, focusing on maintaining control and consistency. The drill can be practiced for a set amount of time or until one player reaches a certain number of successful shots.

Tips: Emphasize the importance of a gentle touch on the ball to keep it low and under control. Focus on consistency rather than power. The goal is to keep the rally going and maintain control.

Third Shot Drop:

Purpose: This drill helps players develop touch and finesse, which are crucial for executing effective drop shots during a game. Here's how you can set up and practice the third shot drop drill:

Setup: Find a pickleball court and divide it into two halves using the centerline. Stand at the non-volley zone (kitchen) line on one side of the court. Your partner should stand at the corresponding position on the other side.

Instructions: Begin the drill by rallying with your partner, hitting cross-court dinks (soft shots) to each other. After a few rallies, initiate the drill by aiming to hit a drop shot just over the net. Your partner should respond by hitting a drop shot back to you, aiming to land it just over the net as well. Continue exchanging drop shots back and forth, focusing on keeping the ball low and placing it close to the net. Aim to hit the drop shot softly with underspin, causing the ball to bounce low and close to the net on your opponent's side.

Tips: Focus on soft hands and a gentle touch when hitting the drop shot. Avoid swinging too hard. Keep your wrist relaxed, and use a short backswing to generate just enough power to clear the net. Aim to hit the drop shot just over the net, allowing it to bounce low and close to the net on your opponent's side.

Volley Practice:

Purpose: Improve your volley skills by volleying with a partner at the net. Focus on control and placement.

Setup: Place cones or markers on each side of the net, on the opponent's side, at various locations (e.g., near the baseline, at mid-court, and close to the net). These will serve as targets for the player. Players start at the non-volley zone (the kitchen).

Instructions: Player A initiates the drill by softly lobbing the ball to player B, who stands at the kitchen line. Player B volleys the ball back to player A, aiming for one of the marked targets. Player A volleys the ball back to player B, who continues to aim for targets on player A's side. Continue rallying back and forth, focusing on hitting the targets with control and accuracy.

Tips: Maintain soft hands and a stable paddle position for better control during volleys, keep a good ready position and stay balanced throughout the drill.

Groundstroke Drills:

Purpose: Focuses on improving your ability to hit consistent and powerful shots from the baseline.

Setup: Stand on opposite baselines (behind the baseline) on either side of the court. Start rallying back and forth using only groundstrokes (forehand and backhand). The goal is to keep the ball in play and maintain a steady rhythm.

Instruction: Focus on technique and pay attention to your footwork, grip, swing technique, and follow-through. Your strokes should be smooth and controlled.

Tips: Aim to hit the ball consistently over the net and within the boundaries of the court. Focus on hitting your shots with the proper amount of power and spin to keep them in play.

Once you feel comfortable with the basic groundstroke rally, you can add variation to the drill by incorporating different types of shots, such as cross-court shots, down-the-line shots, and lobs. As you become more proficient, you can increase the intensity of the rally by hitting the ball harder and faster.

Smash Practice:

Purpose: Aimed to improve your ability to execute powerful overhead shots, commonly known as smashes. Here's a basic smash drill you might consider for practice:

Setup: Players are on either side of the net, typically in pairs.

Instruction: One player (the "feeder") starts the drill by hitting a high lob or "setup" shot to the opposing side of the court. The receiving player then moves into position and executes a smash, aiming to hit the ball downward with power and precision. The objective is to place the smash in a location on the court that makes it difficult for the opposing team to return.

Tips: Vary the objective in many ways to focus on different aspects of the smash, such as accuracy, placement, or power.

Skill Development

Improving your pickleball skills requires a holistic approach that combines dedicated practice, strategic thinking, and physical fitness. First and foremost, practice is the foundation of skill enhancement. Regularly hitting the courts and refining your shots using some or all of the previous drills mentioned helps build muscle memory and precision. Mastering the art of strategic thinking or the ability to make informed decisions and plan your shots and movements on the court is a way to maximize your chances of winning points and, ultimately, the game. Having an understanding of your court positioning and shot selection and anticipating your opponent's moves will give you a significant edge.

Maintaining a high level of fitness is essential for agility, speed, and endurance for skill development on the pickleball court. Engaging in strength and endurance training, as well as cardio exercises as mentioned in previous chapters, can ensure you're in peak physical condition. Here is my advice for skill development in pickleball:

Master the Basics:

- Work on your grip, stance, and basic shots like the dink, drive, and volley.

- Develop a consistent serve that gets you into a favorable position.

Footwork:

- As previously mentioned, footwork is crucial in pickleball. Practice quick lateral movements and positioning to be in the right place on the court.

Strategy:

- Learn the various strategies for singles and doubles play by watching professional players in person or on TV.

- Understand when to be aggressive and when to play defensively.

Shot Variety:

- Develop a range of shots, including lobs, drop shots, and spins.

- Being unpredictable can give you an edge.

Practice Drills:

- Work on drills that focus on specific aspects of your game, such as serving, volleying, or returning.

Partner Play:

- Practice with different partners to adapt to different playing styles and improve your teamwork.

Fitness:

- It may seem obvious, but it is worth the mention and reminder: it is extremely important to maintain good fitness to ensure endurance and quick recovery between points.

Watch and Learn:

- Study professional pickleball matches to pick up techniques and strategies.

Compete and Review:

- Participate in tournaments or friendly matches to apply what you've learned, and review your performance to identify areas for improvement.

Mental Game:

Work on mental toughness, focus, and maintaining a positive attitude on the court.

Seek Coaching:

- Consider taking lessons from a qualified pickleball coach who can provide personalized guidance.

Equipment:

- Invest in quality pickleball paddles (see chapter 7 for pickleball paddle recommendations) and shoes that suit your playing style. Selecting the ideal pair of pickleball shoes is crucial for optimal support, comfort, and performance on the court. I believe that prioritizing support ensures stability and safety during rapid lateral movements inherent to pickleball. Look for shoes with reinforced sidewalls and sturdy midsoles, as they provide the necessary structure to prevent ankle rolling and offer stability during quick changes in direction. I also recommend shoes with integrated arch support to alleviate strain during prolonged play sessions, enhancing overall comfort and reducing the risk of injuries such as plantar fasciitis.

  Comfort is equally paramount in pickleball footwear selection. Opt for shoes with ample cushioning in the midsole and heel areas to absorb impact and minimize fatigue during intense matches. Breathable materials in the upper ensure proper ventilation, keeping feet cool and dry even in warm climates. A snug yet not overly tight fit prevents slippage and blisters that can be painful and inhibit performance. Prioritize shoes with padded collars and tongue for added comfort, which will allow you to concentrate solely on your performance without distractions. Finding the perfect balance between support and comfort leads to enhanced performance and enjoyment on the pickleball court. Adidas, Asics, Nike, and New Balance are great brand options, but do try them on and move around in them in the store or ask the store what their trial period is to ensure you make the best choice.

Game Strategy and Tactics

One of the key strategies in pickleball is the effective placement of shots. You must aim for areas of the court that are difficult for your opponents to reach, forcing them to make errors or weak returns. This involves both accurate serves and precise groundstrokes. The kitchen, a non-volley zone near the net, adds an extra layer of strategy. You need to carefully time your approach to the net and avoid stepping into this zone while hitting volleys, or else you'll lose the point.

Tactics in pickleball also include effective communication and positioning for doubles play. Teamwork and understanding your partner's strengths and weaknesses is crucial. You and your partner must work together to cover the court efficiently, set up winning shots, and anticipate your opponents' moves. Quick reflexes and the ability to adapt to the fast pace are also important tactical skills.

To play at a high level, players must adopt specific tactics during a match. This adaptability is essential to exploit an opponent's weaknesses and respond to changing game dynamics. Whether it's adjusting the pace of play, utilizing dinks and lobs, or executing well-placed shots, the ability to change tactics on the fly is a hallmark of skilled pickleball players. Here are some basic game strategies and tactics to improve your pickleball skills:

Positioning: Positioning in pickleball strategy will help you quickly excel as a dominant player. Effective positioning involves a delicate balance of offense and defense, requiring you to anticipate your opponents' shots while strategically placing them to exploit openings on the court. By staying mindful of court coverage and maintaining a strong net presence, you can control the pace of the game and dictate the flow of play. Whether it's maintaining the kitchen line to control the net or adjusting positioning to counter opponents' shots, strategic placement is the key to success in pickleball.

Serve placement: Serve placement is a crucial aspect of strategy that can dictate the flow of the game. By strategically placing your serves, you can put pressure on your opponents and set yourself up for a strong position in the rally. Whether targeting the sidelines to force difficult returns or aiming for the opponents' weaker side to exploit vulnerabilities, thoughtful serve placement can disrupt your opponents' rhythm and give you the upper hand from the very start. Consistency and variation are key as well. You want to mix up your serves to keep your opponents guessing and prevent them from settling into a comfortable return pattern. Mastering serve placement not only enhances your chances of winning points directly off the serve but also lays the groundwork for controlling the pace and direction of the game.

Dinking: You should prioritize placement shots to exploit weaknesses in your opponents' positioning while maintaining a strong defensive stance to anticipate and counter incoming shots. Utilizing the kitchen line strategically will limit your opponents' opportunities for aggressive plays while maximizing control over the pace of the game. Additionally, effective communication and teamwork with your partner are essential for seamless coordination and capitalizing on scoring opportunities.

Volleying: Mastering the art of volleying can be the key to dominating the game. A successful volley strategy involves quick reflexes, precise positioning, and strategic shot placement. By staying close to the net, you can cut off angles and put pressure on your opponents, forcing them into defensive positions. Communication and teamwork are crucial, especially in doubles play, where partners can cover each other's weaknesses and exploit openings together. Maintaining a low, ready stance and anticipating the opponent's shots are essential elements of effective volleying, allowing you to control the pace of the game and seize opportunities to score points.

Lobbing: The lob can be a strategic weapon when used judiciously. Timing and placement are crucial, and a well-executed lob can force opponents out of position, creating opportunities for offensive plays. However, excessive lobs can also be risky, as they give opponents time to set up for a strong return. Therefore, incorporating lobs into your game plan should be balanced with other shots, such as drives and dinks, to keep opponents guessing and maintain control of the point.

Mastering the lob as part of a multifaceted strategy can elevate your pickleball game to the next level.

Communication: Clear and concise communication between you and your partner ensures seamless coordination on the court, enhancing gameplay and increasing chances of success. Whether it's signaling for who takes the ball, calling out shots, or providing encouragement, constant communication fosters synergy and adaptability. These open lines of communication will help you and your partner anticipate each other's moves, adjust tactics swiftly, and ultimately outmaneuver your opponents to secure victory.

Shot selection: Shot selection can and should be assessed in each situation, considering factors such as court position, opponent placement, and your own strengths and weaknesses. Whether it's a soft dink to force opponents out of position, a powerful drive to exploit an opening, or a well-placed drop shot to catch opponents off guard, the right shot at the right time can change the momentum of a match. Adaptability and precision are key as you constantly analyze the game's dynamics to make split-second decisions that give you the upper hand on the court.

Mind games: The art of mind games can be just as crucial as perfecting your shots. Strategic deception can be a game-changer, keeping opponents on their toes and unsure of your next move. Whether it's disguising your shot direction, feigning a weakness to lure them into a trap, or subtly altering your pace to throw off their rhythm, the psychological aspect of the game is often as intense as the physical. By strategically playing with your opponents' expectations and perceptions, you can gain a significant advantage and control the flow of the match. In pickleball, the mind truly is a powerful weapon on the court.

Aggressive play: Aggressive play in pickleball involves seizing control of the game by putting pressure on your opponents with powerful shots and strategic placement. This style of play often includes attacking the net aggressively, looking for opportunities to volley and smash, and maintaining a strong offensive position on the court. Aim to dictate the pace of the game, forcing your opponents into defensive positions and capitalizing on any weaknesses in their game. By playing aggressively, you can keep your opponents on the defensive, leading to more opportunities to score points and ultimately win the match.

Adaptability: Adaptability is the ability to quickly adjust tactics based on opponents' strengths and weaknesses. Whether it's shifting from offensive to defensive play, altering shot selection to exploit openings, or changing court positioning to cover vulnerabilities, adaptability ensures you stay one step ahead. Flexibility in strategy allows for effective responses to varying game conditions, opponent styles, and unforeseen challenges, ultimately enhancing performance and increasing the chances of victory on the court.

Practice: In the dynamic world of pickleball, where strategy and tactics can make all the difference between victory and defeat, practice emerges as the ultimate cornerstone. Through consistent repetition and refinement, you will not only sharpen your skills but also develop the strategic acumen to adapt to diverse opponents and game scenarios. Practice not only enhances your individual performance but also fortifies the collective strategy of the team. In the arena of pickleball, where split-second decisions determine outcomes, diligent practice remains the linchpin for achieving mastery and unlocking the full potential of your strategic prowess.

CHAPTER 7:

Equipment and Gear

Choosing the Right Paddle

Choosing the right paddle for pickleball is of paramount importance for players of all skill levels. The paddle is not just a piece of equipment; it is an extension of the player's skills and style on the court. There are several components to a paddle's performance, including weight, grip size, shape, and material, that will significantly impact your style of play. For beginners, selecting a paddle that suits your physical attributes and playing style can make the learning curve more manageable and enjoyable. If you are an intermediate player, you will benefit from a paddle that enhances more control and power, allowing you to refine your techniques and skills. And if you are an advanced player, you will rely on a finely tuned paddle to gain a competitive edge that will impact shot accuracy and spin.

The right pickleball paddle can improve your game, prevent injuries, and increase the enjoyment of this sport. Below are several key components and considerations to help you make a better choice for your style and level of play:

Paddle material:

- Composite: Offers a balance of power and control.

- Graphite: Lightweight and provides excellent control.

- Polymer: Known for a softer feel and less vibration.

Weight:

- Light paddles (7.3‑7.8 ounces) offer more control and maneuverability.

- Medium-weight paddles (7.9–8.4 ounces) balance control and power.

- Heavy paddles (8.5+ ounces) provide power but can be less maneuverable.

Grip Size:

- Choose a grip size that feels comfortable and allows you to maintain a relaxed grip during play.

Paddle Shape:

- Wide-body paddles offer a larger sweet spot and more power.

- Narrow-body paddles provide better control and accuracy.

Playing Style:

- Power players: Look for paddles with a larger hitting surface and heavier weight.

- Control players: Opt for lighter, narrower paddles with a smaller sweet spot.

Noise Level:

- Some venues have noise restrictions, so consider a quieter paddle if needed.

Price:

- Set a budget and look for paddles that offer the best features within that range.

Test Different Paddles:

- If possible, try out different paddles to find the one that suits your style and comfort best.

Reviews and Recommendations:

- Research online reviews and seek recommendations from experienced players.

When making the final decision to purchase a pickleball paddle, here are three popular online platforms where you can find a variety of pickleball paddles for all levels:

Amazon: Amazon offers a vast selection of pickleball paddles from various brands, including best-sellers like Franklin, ONIX, PickleballCentral, and more. You can easily filter your search based on factors like price range, ratings, and specific features to find the paddle that suits your preferences. www.amazon.com.

PickleballCentral: PickleballCentral is a dedicated online store specializing in all things pickleball. They offer a wide range of paddles from beginner to advanced levels, along with detailed product descriptions and customer reviews to help you make an informed decision. PickleballCentral also provides expert advice and guidance for selecting the right paddle. www.pickleballcentral.com

Dick's Sporting Goods: Dick's Sporting Goods is a popular destination for sports equipment, including pickleball paddles. They carry a diverse selection of paddles from leading brands like HEAD, Wilson, and Gamma. Their website allows you to browse various options and filter results based on price, brand, and customer ratings. www.dickssportinggoods.com

Footwear and Apparel

When it comes to footwear and apparel, it is often a personal choice based on style or loyalty to a brand. I am a believer of fashion over function. However, for the game of pickleball, this rule might not apply. It is important to choose athletic shoes with good lateral support and grip to allow for quick movements on the court and apparel that will be comfortable, flexible, and moisture-wicking. Popular brands like ASICS, Nike, New Balance, Head, Wilson, and Franklin offer pickleball-specific shoes and apparel.

There isn't a definitive "best" place to buy pickleball shoes online, as it can depend on factors like your location, shoe preferences, budget, and availability. However, here are two popular and reputable online retailers where you can often find a good selection of pickleball shoes:

Amazon: Amazon offers a wide variety of pickleball shoes from various brands, including popular options like ASICS, Nike, Adidas, and more. Read customer reviews, compare prices, and find competitive deals. I recommend checking the seller's reputation and return policy before making a purchase. www.amazon.com

Zappos: Zappos is known for its extensive selection of shoes, including pickleball shoes. They offer a user-friendly interface, detailed product descriptions, and excellent customer service. Zappos also has a generous return policy, allowing you to return items within 365 days of purchase for a full refund, making it a popular choice for online shoe shopping. www.zappos.com

Maintenance and Care

Caring for your gear in pickleball is essential to maintain its integrity for peak performance, longevity, and safety. Well-maintained equipment, including your paddle and balls, ensures that you can play at your best. A clean and undamaged paddle enables precise shots and power, contributing to your overall gameplay. Regular maintenance also extends the lifespan of your gear, saving you money in the long run. Properly maintained equipment is not only safe but also consistent, allowing you to rely on its performance and maintain your playing style. By following regular maintenance practices and manufacturer guidelines, you can enhance your game and make your investment in pickleball gear more cost-efficient. Here are some of my suggestions:

Pickleball Paddles:

- Wipe the surface of your paddle with a damp cloth after each game to remove dirt and sweat.

- Use edge guard tape to protect the edges of your paddle from chips and dings.

- Store your paddle in a padded bag when not in use to prevent damage.

- Don't expose your paddle to extreme heat or cold, as it can affect the materials.

Pickleball Balls:

- Regularly inspect pickleball balls for cracks or deformities. Discard damaged balls.

- Clean your pickleball balls with a damp cloth to remove dirt and grime.

- Store pickleball balls in a cool, dry place to prevent warping.

- Rotate your ball usage to ensure even wear among a set.

Court Maintenance:

- Keep the pickleball court clean and free of debris.

- Sweep the court surface to remove loose dirt and leaves.

- Repair any cracks or damage on the court surface promptly.

Footwear:

- Wear proper court shoes with non-marking soles to protect the court surface and provide good traction.

Nets and Posts:

- Inspect and tighten the net and posts regularly to ensure they are in good condition.

Cultivating this habit of caring for and maintaining your gear and equipment not only demonstrates respect for your gear but also reflects a commitment to personal improvement and longevity in the sport.

CHAPTER 8:

Longevity in Pickleball

Age-Related Considerations

Age-related considerations in pickleball play a crucial role in shaping the dynamics of the game. Pickleball is lauded because it is accessible to people of all ages, but players are required to adapt their strategies and gameplay as they get older. Younger players may rely on their agility and speed to cover the court efficiently, while older individuals may prioritize precision and strategic placement to compensate for reduced mobility. As mentioned in chapter 5, the risk of injuries, such as strains and sprains, tends to increase with age, necessitating careful warm-ups, adequate conditioning, and possibly a modified playing style to minimize the chances of injury. Nevertheless, the social and physical benefits of playing pickleball can be enjoyed throughout one's life, making it a sport that will continue to thrive among players of varying age groups. Here are some general age-related guidelines that I believe will keep you playing at peak performance at any age:

Young Players (Under 40):

- Focus on building and maintaining strength, agility, and speed.

- Emphasize skill development and strategy.

- Injury prevention through proper warm-up and cool-down routines.

Middle-Aged Players (40-60):

- Maintain a balance between fitness and skill development.

- Pay attention to joint health and flexibility.

- Consider using the appropriate equipment and footwear to reduce strain.

Senior Players (60+):

- Prioritize flexibility and joint mobility.

- Play at a pace that matches your fitness level and avoid overexertion.

- Use paddles that are easy on the joints and provide control.

- Adapt your playing style to reduce the risk of injury.

Training for Seniors

Training for seniors in pickleball is a fantastic way to promote both physical fitness and social engagement among the older generation. Pickleball is one of the most ideal sports for seniors due to its low-impact nature and accessibility. Seniors can enjoy the benefits of improved balance, coordination, agility, hand-eye coordination, and cardiovascular health while minimizing the risk of injury. Tailored training programs for seniors should focus on building fundamental skills such as proper footwork, change of direction, reaction drills, strength, and recovery.

In addition to the physical benefits, the social aspect of pickleball training for seniors fosters a sense of community and camaraderie, providing a wonderful opportunity for friendships to flourish on the court. Whether they're picking up a paddle for the first time or honing their skills, if you are a senior, you can savor the joy of pickleball while maintaining an active and fulfilling lifestyle. Below is a basic training program outline for seniors:

Sample Peak Performance Program for Seniors

Warm-Up:

- Start with light aerobic activities like walking or stationary cycling to warm up the muscles.

- Follow with gentle joint mobility exercises to improve flexibility.

Basic Pickleball Skills:

- Practice the basic rules and techniques of pickleball, including serving, forehand and backhand shots, and court positioning.

Low-Intensity Drills:

- Begin with slow-paced drills to practice control and accuracy.

- Focus on improving hand-eye coordination and footwork.

Cardiovascular Exercise:

- Incorporate light cardiovascular exercises to improve endurance, like brisk walking or easy jogging.

Doubles Play:

- Emphasize the importance of teamwork and communication when playing doubles.

- Practice positioning and covering the court effectively.

Balance and Agility Training:

- Include balance exercises to prevent falls, and agility drills to improve on-court mobility.

Strength Training:

- Use resistance bands or light weights for strength training to maintain muscle mass and bone density.

Cool Down and Stretching:

- End each session with a cool-down period and gentle stretching to reduce muscle soreness and improve flexibility.

Social Play:

- Promote the social aspect of pickleball, as it's a great way for seniors to connect with others and stay active.

Safety Precautions:

- Stay hydrated, wear appropriate footwear, and use sun protection when playing outdoors.

Staying Competitive at Any Age

To maintain competitiveness, you must adopt a multifaceted approach that encompasses both physical and mental aspects. Cultivate a healthy lifestyle from the inside out beginning with proper nutrition and regular exercise to fuel and strengthen the body and enhance cognitive function. Equally important is adequate rest and relaxation, as sufficient sleep allows for proper recovery and promotes mental clarity.

Continuous learning and skill development are essential for staying ahead and competing at peak levels. Keep abreast of trends and advancements and hone relevant skills to ensure you remain adaptable and capable of meeting the evolving demands of the sport and your abilities. Further, foster a growth mindset to help facilitate resilience in the face of challenges, allowing you to view setbacks as opportunities for learning and improvement rather than obstacles.

Lastly, staying competitive at any age requires a commitment to continuous learning and improvement. Embracing new techniques, staying updated on rule changes and innovations in equipment, and participating in clinics, workshops, or competitions provide opportunities for growth and development as a pickleball player. By integrating physical conditioning, mental resilience, strategic acumen, and a dedication to lifelong learning, players can maintain their competitive edge and excel in pickleball at any age.Staying competitive in pickleball as you age is not only possible but can also be incredibly rewarding. Pickleball is a sport that can be enjoyed by individuals of all ages and fitness levels, and as you get older, there are several strategies you can employ to maintain your competitive edge on the court.

Age should never be a barrier to staying competitive in pickleball. While it's true that physical abilities may change with time, the sport offers numerous opportunities for you to adapt and excel regardless of age.

CHAPTER 9

The Pickleball Community

Finding Playing Partners

Finding playing partners for pickleball can be an enjoyable and social endeavor. Pickleball enthusiasts often connect with others who share their passion for the sport through various avenues. The quest for pickleball playing partners not only enhances your game but also fosters lasting friendships. Finding playing partners for pickleball can be a fun way to enjoy the sport. Here are some places to find playing partners:

Local pickleball clubs: Join a local pickleball club or association. They often have scheduled play times and can help you connect with others looking for partners.

Social media: Look for pickleball groups on platforms like Facebook or Meetup. You can often find people in your area who are looking for playing partners or events.

Pickleball apps: There are dedicated pickleball apps, like PicklePlay, that can help you find nearby players and events.

Online forums: Participate in pickleball forums and discussion boards. You can post that you're looking for playing partners in your area.

Community centers: Many community centers and sports facilities offer pickleball. You can often find players there and connect with them.

Local pickleball courts: If there are public pickleball courts in your area, simply showing up and asking people if they'd like to play is a good way to find partners.

Pickleball tournaments: Attend local pickleball tournaments. You'll likely meet players of various skill levels who may be interested in playing.

Friends and family: Introduce friends or family members to pickleball. They could become your regular playing partners.

Communication is key to any good relationship, including the people you play pickleball with. Therefore, communicate your skill level and availability to potential partners to ensure a good match. Whether you're a beginner or an advanced player, there are likely others in your area looking for pickleball partners.

Staying Engaged in Pickleball

Staying engaged in pickleball requires a combination of enthusiasm, practice, and a positive mindset. To maintain your passion for this fast-paced and exciting game, it's important to keep a few key principles in mind. First, set clear goals for your pickleball journey. Whether it's improving your serve, perfecting your dink shots, or winning more matches, having specific objectives can help you stay motivated. Second, vary your playing experience by participating in different formats, such as singles, doubles, or mixed doubles, to keep the game fresh and challenging. Finally, engage with the pickleball community. Joining a local club or participating in tournaments can provide you with a sense of camaraderie and friendly competition that fuels your passion.

Continue learning and refining your skills through practice, drills, and watching professional players. Staying engaged in pickleball is about embracing the sport's continuous evolution and finding joy in the journey of improvement. Here are some recommendations to help you stay engaged:

Practice regularly: Regular practice is essential for staying engaged in pickleball, as it not only improves skill level but also fosters a deeper connection to the game. Consistent practice sessions help maintain muscle memory, refine technique, and enhance strategic thinking, making each game more rewarding and enjoyable.

Vary opponents: Facing a variety of opponents is crucial for staying engaged in pickleball, as it challenges players to adapt their strategies and tactics. Playing against different styles and skill levels enhances one's overall game, fosters versatility, and keeps the experience dynamic and stimulating. It also offers opportunities for learning and growth, ensuring continued interest and enthusiasm for the sport.

Learn new techniques: Continue to learn and incorporate new techniques and shots into your game.

Focus on strategy: Prioritize strategy by anticipating your opponent's moves and adapting your gameplay accordingly.

Focusing on strategic plays not only keeps you mentally involved but also enhances your overall performance on the court.

Set goals: Establish specific goals to work toward, whether it's improving your serve, winning a certain number of points, or mastering a particular shot.

Stay physically fit: Regular exercise and conditioning are essential for maintaining your energy and focus during matches.

Watch and analyze: Actively watch your opponent's movements and analyze their patterns and tendencies. By observing and assessing their gameplay, you can strategically adjust your approach, leading to a more dynamic and engaging match experience.

Socialize: Engage in conversations with fellow players during breaks or after matches to foster a sense of community and camaraderie on the pickleball court. Socializing not only enhances your enjoyment of the game but also provides opportunities for learning and building lasting connections with other players.

Have fun: Ultimately, keep in mind that pickleball is a fun and enjoyable sport, so focus on having a good time on the court!

Overcoming Challenges

Like overcoming any challenge in sports or life, pickleball requires a combination of skill development, strategy, and a positive mindset. One key aspect is improving your technique through practice and proper coaching. Work on your paddle control, footwork, and shot selection to become a more well-rounded player.

As mentioned above, focus on new strategies. Learn to anticipate your opponent's moves, adapt to different playing styles, and make effective shot choices. Maintaining a positive attitude and staying focused during matches can also help you overcome challenges. Pickleball can be physically demanding, so ensure you are in good shape and practice regularly to build your endurance and agility.

Don't be afraid to seek advice from more experienced players and be open to constructive criticism. By continually honing your skills and maintaining a determined mindset, you can tackle and conquer challenges in pickleball.

Conclusion

My goal in writing this book was to give you a comprehensive guide to the sport of pickleball, from its history and rules to essential techniques and strategies. I hope that the knowledge and insights shared within these pages have not only enhanced your understanding of the game but also kindled your passion for this exciting and rapidly growing sport. As you embark on your pickleball journey, remember that success in this game, like in life, often requires dedication, practice, and a love for the thrill of competition. Whether you're a beginner looking to master the basics or an experienced player seeking to elevate your game, may this book serve as a valuable resource and source of inspiration as you continue to enjoy the game of pickleball. Keep paddling, keep learning, and most importantly, keep having fun on the courts.

Pickleball is a fantastic choice for improving your health and fitness! It's a low-impact sport that's easy on your joints and offers a great cardiovascular workout. Playing regularly can enhance your agility, balance, and coordination. Plus, it's a fun way to socialize and stay active. Keep pursuing pickleball. Your body and mind will thank you!

Resources for Ongoing Learning and Improvement

Improving your pickleball skills requires ongoing learning and practice. Here are some resources I recommend to help you with your pickleball journey:

Online videos and tutorials: Websites like YouTube have a plethora of pickleball tutorials, drills, and match analysis videos. Channels like *Pickleball Channel* and *PrimeTime Pickleball* are great places to start. Visit www.pickleballpowerbook.com for videos and other programs to help you achieve the level of success you deserve.

Pickleball clinics and camps: Look for local or regional pickleball clinics and camps. These events often bring in experienced coaches and players who can provide hands-on instruction.

Books: There are several books dedicated to pickleball strategy and techniques. *Smart Pickleball* by Prem Carnot and *Pickleball Fundamentals* by Mary Littlewood are popular choices.

Online courses: Websites like Udemy and Skillshare offer online pickleball courses that cover various aspects of the game, from basics to advanced strategies.

Pickleball forums and communities: Join online pickleball forums and communities where you can discuss strategy, ask questions, and learn from other players. Websites like Pickleball Forum and Facebook groups dedicated to pickleball are good places to start.

Mobile apps: There are mobile apps designed to help you improve your pickleball skills. They offer drills, score tracking, and video analysis. Check out apps like Pickleball Tutor and Pickleball Coach.

Private coaching: Consider hiring a private coach for one-on-one instruction. They can provide personalized feedback and tailored training programs to address your specific needs.

Tournaments and competitions: Participating in pickleball tournaments can be a great way to learn from more experienced players. You can watch and play against top-level competitors.

Equipment reviews: Stay updated on the latest pickleball equipment and read reviews to find the best paddles, shoes, and gear that suit your playing style.

Podcasts: Some pickleball podcasts, like *The Pickleball Kitchen* and *Pickleball Fire*, feature interviews with top players and coaches, providing valuable insights.

Local clubs: Join a local pickleball club or association to connect with fellow players, find playing partners, and participate in organized events.

Online courses: Enroll in online courses dedicated to pickleball. Some platforms, like Udemy and Skillshare, offer courses on various aspects of the game.

Appendices

Glossary of Pickleball Terms

around-the-post: A shot that goes around the net post and lands in the opponent's court.

backspin: A type of spin applied to the ball, causing it to rotate backward, making it bounce higher.

baseline: The back boundary of the court.

dink: A soft, controlled shot typically hit close to the net.

double bounce rule: In doubles play, the ball must bounce once on each side before players can start volleying it.

drive: A powerful shot aimed to clear the net and land deep in the opponent's court.

erne shot: A shot where the player quickly moves to the non-volley zone line to hit a ball that's close to the net.

fault: An error that results in the loss of a point, such as a serve that doesn't clear the net.

kitchen: Also known as the *non-volley zone*, it's the area close to the net where players are not allowed to volley the ball.

let: A serve that hits the net but still lands in the proper service court and is replayed.

non-volley zone line: The line at the edge of the kitchen, which marks the boundary where players can't volley the ball.

pickleball court: The playing area, which is smaller than a tennis court, typically twenty feet wide and forty-four feet long.

pickleball grip: The way players hold the paddle, with popular grips including the eastern, western, and continental grips.

pickleball paddle: The equipment used to hit the ball, usually made of composite materials or wood.

poach: When one player in a doubles team crosses over to hit a ball that's on their partner's side.

rally: A sequence of shots exchanged by players during a point.

side-out: When the serving team loses the serve, usually due to a fault, and the opposing team takes over serving.

topspin: A type of spin applied to the ball, causing it to rotate forward, making it drop more quickly.

These are what I would consider the most important pickleball terms to get you started. The game has its own unique vocabulary, and learning these terms can enhance your understanding and enjoyment of the sport.

Sample Peak Performance Training Plan

General Peak Performance Training Plan

Week 1–2: Fundamentals and Conditioning

Day 1:

- Warm-up (10 minutes)

- Forehand and backhand drills (20 minutes)

- Serve practice (10 minutes)

- Footwork and agility drills (15 minutes)

- Cool down (5 minutes)

Day 2:

- Warm-up (10 minutes)

- Dinking drills (20 minutes)

- Volleys and smashes (15 minutes)

- Cardio and endurance training (20 minutes)

- Cool down (5 minutes)

Day 3: Rest or light activity

Day 4:

- Warm-up (10 minutes)

- Strategy and positioning (20 minutes)

- Game simulation (15 minutes)

- Cross-court shots and lobs (20 minutes)

- Cool down (5 minutes)

Day 5:

- Warm-up (10 minutes)

- Practicing third shot drops (15 minutes)

- Mini-tournaments (20 minutes)

- Strength training (20 minutes)

- Cool down (5 minutes)

Day 6: Rest or light activity

Day 7:

- Warm-up (10 minutes)

- Review and refine various shots (20 minutes)

- Match play (30 minutes)

- Cool down (5 minutes)

Week 3–4: Advanced Skills and Match Play

Day 1–4:

- Warm-up (10 minutes)

- Intensive drills focusing on specific weaknesses (20 minutes)

- Match play (30 minutes)

- Cool down (5 minutes)

Day 5:

- Warm–up (10 minutes)

- Singles match practice (30 minutes)

- Doubles strategy and communication (20 minutes)

- Strength and agility training (20 minutes)

- Cool down (5 minutes)

Day 6: Rest or light activity

Day 7:

- Warm-up (10 minutes)

- Competitive match play (45 minutes)

- Cool down (5 minutes)

Week 5–6: Pre-Tournament Preparation

Day 1-3:

- Warm-up (10 minutes)

- Fine-tuning shots and strategy (30 minutes)

- Tournament-style practice matches (45 minutes)

- Cool down (5 minutes)

Day 4: Rest

Day 5:

- Warm-up (10 minutes)

- Review tournament strategy and mental preparation (30 minutes)

- Light practice (20 minutes)

- Visualization and relaxation (15 minutes)

- Cool down (5 minutes)

Day 6: Rest

Day 7: Tournament Day

Remember to adjust the plan to your individual needs and skill level, and gradually increase the intensity of your training as you progress. It's also essential to include proper nutrition and rest in your overall training routine.

Peak Performance Sample Workouts:

Beginner Pickleball Player

A workout for a beginner pickleball player should focus on improving agility, strength, endurance, and balance. Pickleball requires quick lateral movements, explosive power, and good cardiovascular fitness. Here's a sample workout plan:

Warm-up (5–10 minutes):

- Start with light cardio, such as jogging or jumping jacks, to raise your heart rate.

- Perform dynamic stretches for your legs, arms, and shoulders.

- Warm up your pickleball strokes by hitting some balls against a wall or with a partner.

Strength Training (2–3 times per week):

- **Squats:** 3 sets of 10–12 reps to build leg strength for powerful movements on the court.

- **Lunges:** 3 sets of 10 reps per leg to improve balance and leg strength.

- **Push-ups:** 3 sets of 10–15 reps for upper body strength.

- **Planks:** Hold for 30–60 seconds to strengthen your core.

- **Dumbbell rows:** 3 sets of 10–12 reps to work on your back and shoulder muscles.

Cardiovascular Training (3–4 times per week):

- Incorporate cardio exercises like running, cycling, or high-intensity interval training (HIIT) to build endurance and improve your ability to cover the court.

Agility and Footwork (2–3 times per week):

- Set up agility ladder drills or cone drills to improve your footwork and lateral movement.

- Practice side-to-side shuffling, quick direction changes, and explosive starts.

Pickleball-Specific Skills Training (2–3 times per week):

- Work on your serves, returns, and volleys with a partner or against a wall.

- Practice dinking, third shot drops, and smashes to improve your technique.

Balance and Core (2 times per week):

- Include exercises like single-leg squats, balance board exercises, and stability ball work to enhance your balance and core strength.

Cooldown (5–10 minutes):

- Finish your workout with static stretching to improve flexibility and reduce the risk of injury.

Rest and Recovery:

- Ensure you have rest days to allow your body to recover and prevent overtraining.

Nutrition:

- Maintain a well-balanced diet to support your training and performance. Focus on lean proteins, complex carbohydrates, and healthy fats. Stay hydrated.

Remember to adjust the intensity and volume of your workouts based on your current fitness level and any specific goals you may have. It's also a good idea to consult with a fitness trainer or coach to create a more personalized workout plan tailored to your needs and abilities.

Intermediate Pickleball Player

A well-rounded workout routine for an intermediate pickleball player should focus on improving balance, strength, endurance, agility, and flexibility. At the intermediate level, pickleball requires quick bursts of energy, lateral movement, and hand-eye coordination. Here's a sample workout plan:

Warm-up (5–10 minutes):

- Start with light cardio, like jogging in place or jumping jacks.

- Follow with dynamic stretches for the legs, arms, and torso.

Strength Training (2–3 times a week):

- Single-leg squats: 3 sets of 10–12 reps

- Push-up with rotation: 3 sets of 10–12 reps

- Side plank with rotation: 3 sets of 30–60 seconds

- Single-leg dumbbell rows: 3 sets of 10–12 reps (each arm)

- Lateral lunges: 3 sets of 10–12 reps (each leg)

Agility and Speed (2 times a week):

- Ladder drills: Perform ladder drills to improve footwork and agility.

- Cone drills: Set up a series of cones and practice moving quickly in different directions.

- Suicides: Sprint back and forth between two markers, gradually increasing the distance.

Cardiovascular Conditioning (3–4 times a week):

Incorporate cardio exercises like running, cycling, or interval training to improve endurance and cardiovascular health. Aim for at least 30 minutes of moderate- to high-intensity cardio.

Pickleball-Specific Training (2–3 times a week):

Play pickleball regularly to hone your skills, improve your reactions, and practice different shots.

Flexibility and Mobility (3–4 times a week):

Stretch major muscle groups to maintain flexibility and reduce the risk of injury. Focus on your legs, arms, shoulders, and back.

Cooldown (5–10 minutes):

Finish your workout with static stretches for the major muscle groups.

Nutrition and Hydration:

Stay properly hydrated before, during, and after workouts.

Consume a balanced diet with a focus on lean proteins, complex carbohydrates, and healthy fats to support your energy needs and muscle recovery.

Rest and Recovery:

Ensure you get adequate rest to allow your body to recover and repair itself.

Remember to listen to your body, and if you have any underlying health conditions or concerns, it's a good idea to consult with a healthcare professional before starting a new workout routine. Additionally, consider working with a fitness trainer or coach to tailor your routine to your specific needs and goals as a pickleball player.

Advanced Pickleball Player

Advanced pickleball players should focus on coordinating movements that improve total body strength, agility, and power. Here's a sample workout routine:

Warmup (10–15 minutes):

- Light jogging or brisk walking to increase heart rate.

- Arm circles and leg swings to loosen up the joints.

- Dynamic stretches for the upper and lower body.

Speed, Agility, Quickness (SAQ)(5 min)

- Jump rope – 1 min

- Speed ladder – in/in/out/out, in/in/out, Ali Shuffle – 1 min

- Jump rope – 1 min

- Speed Ladder – in/in/out/out, in/in/out, Ali Shuffle – 1 min

- Jump rope – 1 min

Strength Training (3–4 times a week):

- Deadlifts: 3 sets of 10–12 reps, 60–90% or 1 rep max, rest 1–2 min between sets

- Pullups: 3 sets of 6–12 reps, rest 1–2 min between sets

- Bicycle crunch: 3 sets of 30–60 seconds, rest 1 min between sets

- Ice skaters: 3 sets of 30–60 seconds, rest 1 min between sets

- Squat jumps: 3 sets of 10–12 reps, rest 30 seconds between sets

- Standing long jump: 3 sets of 10–12 reps, rest 30 seconds between sets

Pickleball-Specific Drills (15–20 minutes):

- Practice your pickleball skills. This can include hitting against a wall, partner drills, and simulated games. Work on your dinking, volleying, and transitioning between different shots.

Cooldown and Stretching (10-15 minutes):

- Finish your workout with foam rolling and static stretches for the major muscle groups.

Hydration and Nutrition:

- Stay properly hydrated before, during, and after workouts.

- Consume a balanced diet with a focus on lean proteins, complex carbohydrates, and healthy fats to support your energy needs and muscle recovery.

Overtraining can lead to injury. Remember that this is just a sample workout plan. Adjust the frequency and intensity based on your fitness level and personal goals. It's also a good idea to consult with a fitness professional or a coach to tailor your workout routine to your specific needs as a pickleball player.